# Friendship

# Friendship

## *AN EXPOSÉ*

Joseph Epstein

Houghton Mifflin Company

BOSTON · NEW YORK

2006

For information about permission to reproduce selections
from this book, write to Permissions, Houghton Mifflin Company,
215 Park Avenue South, New York, New York 10003.

Visit our Web site: www.houghtonmifflinbooks.com.

*Library of Congress Cataloging-in-Publication Data*
Epstein, Joseph, date.
Friendship : an exposé / Joseph Epstein.
p. cm.
Includes bibliographical references and index.
ISBN-13: 978-0-618-34149-8
ISBN-10: 0-618-34149-8
1. Epstein, Joseph, date. — Friends and associates.
2. Friendship. 3. Friendship in literature. I. Title.
HM1161.E67 2006
302.3'4 — dc22    2005020059

Printed in the United States of America

QUM 10 9 8 7 6 5 4 3 2 1

*To Arnie Glass*

A smart and good guy — and a friend

The only rose without a thorn is friendship.

—FORTUNE COOKIE

Not a few things about friendship are matters of debate.

—ARISTOTLE, *Nichomachean Ethics*

# Contents

# *Foreword*

This is a book about friendship, its pleasures, complications, and manifold contradictions. The idea for writing the book was given to me, appropriately enough, by a friend, a sociologist and former bookseller in Evanston named Arnie Glass. "You ought to write a book about friendship," Arnie said to me one afternoon over coffee. "It's a subject about which no one has told anything like the full story."

What, I wondered, might the full story be? I had sensed my own friendships becoming more complex the older I had grown. Friendship had long since ceased to be the free-and-easy matter it once seemed. While I had many friends whom I considered dear to me, friendship itself was rarely any longer quite the simple, pleasurable thing it was when I was a boy and young man; nor was it any more at the center of my life. Why? What, if anything, had replaced it? What, exactly, was going on? What was the full story?

A book on a grand general subject like friendship can gain from having an argument or overriding point to make. When I began writing this book I had no such argument to make. But that seemed to me all right. Why write a book whose argument and conclusion one knew in advance? Still, it took a long time for my argument—thesis, case, call it what you will—to emerge. During this period, I often felt like the composer William Walton, who, having been commissioned to write a Theme and Variations, remarked to a friend that he had written all the variations but hadn't yet found the theme.

The first thing I noted, with much relief, is that there is no great book on friendship — no single work that I would have to accommodate or with which I would have to argue. The best thing on the subject was written more than 2,300 years ago, in the twenty-five or so pages devoted to friendship in Aristotle's *Nichomachean Ethics.* Cicero's *De Amicitia,* composed three hundred years later, fills in and fleshes out Aristotle in useful ways. And Montaigne's sixteenth-century essay "On Friendship" records a great friendship — his own with a slightly older contemporary — in an impressive if oddly incomplete manner, along the way remarking on the general nature of friendship.

More recently, lots of therapy-minded books on friendship have appeared, freighted with psychobabble (much soft talk about caring and sharing and nurturing and being there for you and the rest of it), usually written by people whose last names seem to end in the letters Ph.D. These books are about how to make more and better friends, how to get over broken friendships, some offering to tell one "why men and women are indeed from the same planet" or that "friendship brings with it a power to shape our lives." Invariably, these manuals are filled with anecdotes and case studies that reek of low invention and high artificiality. Skimming these books, I realized that the last thing I wanted to write was another how-to book. I don't, after all, know how to master the art of friendship, and I have very little advice to give anyone, on this subject or any other. As it would turn out, what I wrote may be something closer to a how-*not*-to book.

Nor, I was to discover, is there a theory of friendship. Plato, in *Lysis,* his dialogue on friendship, throws up his hands even at defining what a friend is, ending the dialogue by having Socrates say: "For our hearers will carry away the report that though we conceive ourselves to be friends with each other . . . we have not as yet been able to discover what we mean by a friend." Once one allows that friendships exist outside biological ties, everyone is left to define friendship on his or her own.

Perhaps the closest thing to a theory of friendship comes from Sigmund Freud. But Freudian doctrines, if truly believed, would just about eliminate friendship altogether. Eroticizing everything, as is their wont, Freudians find that much close male friendship is at its core homoerotic, while the notion of male-female friends outside sexual interest is generally inconceivable to Freudians, who not so secretly believe that all men wish to do with women is jump their bones.

One of the things I concluded during the writing of my book is that where there is sex, there is not friendship; something else is involved — perhaps many other things — but not friendship. Later in this book I take up the matter of friendship within marriage, and husbands and wives obviously make love. But I would contend that real friendship between husbands and wives sets in after courtship is done, when responsibility (for children and other things) deepens feeling, and appreciation extends well beyond romantic interest.

If I believed in Freud, I could not have written a book on friendship, because friendship doesn't quite exist for Freudians; sexual appetite, evident or obscured, washes it away. Fortunately I do not believe in Freud. In fact, I have come to believe instead that Freudian psychoanalysts, like Germany after World War II, ought to be made to pay reparations to their poor patient-victims.

Without a theory, then, and without any great books about friendship to argue with or revise, what was there to be said about the subject? I could always say that friendship is a damn fine thing, that friends are, *you know,* very "special," but I fear that Hallmark beat me to that particular punch. I didn't wish to go the other way, to say that friendship is a nightmare of obligation and boredom, because, though obligation and boredom can sometimes be a part of friendship, I took too much pleasure from too many friends to believe that. But I did feel that something had changed in the nature of my feelings about friendship and in my relations with many of my friends — and I suspected that I was not alone in these feelings.

I decided to write a book on friendship based in good part on my own experience. The danger here, of course, is that of solipsism, which means, literally, "only-oneselfism," or the belief that oneself is the only existent, and therefore significant, being in the world. When the solipsist gets a cold, he feels the

World Health Organization should be notified; when the solipsist can't find a Kleenex, he blames it on capitalist methods of distribution. But the better solipsistic writers, from Rousseau and Ben Franklin on up to our day, have believed, as I believe, that their uniqueness is only a more intense and public version of your, our readers', uniqueness. When I write about my friendships in this book — many sweet and strong, some burdensome and troubling — I trust that they will also say something about your own friendships.

At times during the writing of this book I felt as if I were writing, along with a general inquiry into a very complex subject, something approaching my autobiography. My friends will recognize themselves in these pages (though they are for the most part not mentioned by name), some to their pleasure, some to their chagrin, and a few to their strong distaste. I hope that, after many of them have read it, I am left with a sufficient number of friends, as the English say, to see me out. I don't claim this is a courageous book, but it is, I fear, rather a reckless one.

I have long had a knack for making friends. If anything, as this book will show, I may have made too many friends, though I continue to count on a small number of them for pleasure, shared interests, and my own continuing education. But friendship, I found in my seventh decade, was no longer the easy pleasure it once was. Often it had come to seem weighed down by a sense of obligation, enforced tolerance, stupefying boredom. The question, of course, is whether this was merely me or whether something had happened to change the nature of friendship. No one will be much surprised when I say that I favor the latter cause.

Once the idea of writing a book on the subject was presented to me, I began to feel that something about the nature of friendship was undergoing change. It also seemed to me that friendship had for too long been idealized, putting unreasonable pressure on friends, and that people — myself among them — didn't wish to acknowledge the immense complications inherent in even the closest of friendships.

Friendships have become more complicated. The changed status of women has in turn radically changed the nature of

many kinds of friendships: between husbands and wives, between men and women, among women themselves. Technology
— through sophisticated telephone systems, easy-access long
distance, and e-mail — has brought friendships into bloom that
might never have been planted thirty or so years ago. What one
wants from — and is willing to give to — friends feels different
than it once did. The standard of what constitutes a genuine
friend has, I believe, been altered. In the pages that follow I attempt to elucidate, elaborate on, and formulate what I take to be
the nature of these changes among American men and women
in the twenty-first century.

For a good writer, there is only one measure of success, and
that is found in his honoring the complexity and richness of his
subject while telling his story in a lucid way. I hope I have
achieved this, and that in doing so to have captured some of
what Arnie Glass had in mind when he spoke of the full story
about friendship.

# Friendship

# 1

✦

# *A Little Taxonomy*
# *of Friends*

T HE BEAUTY OF THE WORD "friend" is that it's so ambiguous," wrote Miss Manners in one of her columns. I take Miss Manners's meaning, though ambiguity is not necessarily a beautiful quality for someone who is attempting to understand what friendship is and how it works, and at book length no less. How much better if the meaning, implications, and significance of the word were nicely locked into a firm and easy definition! Alas, they aren't, and perhaps never will be.

Friendship is the strongest of relationships not bound by or hostage to biology, which is to say, blood. It is, in this sense, as C. S. Lewis writes in *The Four Loves,* "the least *natural* of loves; the least instinctive, organic, biological, gregarious and necessary." As Lewis goes on to point out, we can breed without friendship and carry on existence without it. Friendship does not arise out of necessity, but out of preference. Unlike our family, which we have no say in choosing, our friendships are based almost entirely on personal selection. "God's apology," the English essayist Hugh Kingsmill amusingly called friends; by which he meant that, by way of apology, and to make amends to us for the families He has burdened us with, God has also supplied us with friends.

The breadth of meanings the word "friend" takes in is such

that all one can safely say through definition is that a friend is someone one likes and wishes to see again, though I can think of exceptions and qualifications even to this innocuous formulation. Rather than attempt to define "friend" straightaway, perhaps I do better to begin by distinguishing between the kinds and degrees of friendship.

The first necessary distinction is that between a friend and an acquaintance. Dictionaries aren't of much help here either. An acquaintance, I should say, is someone you know, may even have known for a long while, but almost never plan to meet, unless for some very specific reason. He or she may be someone pleasing enough to encounter — on the street, at a party or professional function, even in a hospital — but one generally does so with a slight element of surprise. A relationship with an acquaintance doesn't postulate a future. You may or may not meet again, no obligation on either side, nothing owed but recognition and civility. You might dislike, in fact despise, an acquaintance, and do so with a clear conscience, something one is not permitted to do with a person one claims to call a friend. Yet there are some who prefer acquaintances to friends, as does the narrator of Julian Fellowes's recent novel *Snobs*, who remarks that he much prefers acquaintances over friends, for they offer more variety and require so much less in the way of participation and obligation, leaving one's life less clogged with human complication.

"Comrade" was a word much in vogue under Communism, which tried to foist equality even on friendship by making all men and women equally one's friend in the forthcoming (it hasn't quite arrived yet) just society. But in the social sense friendship isn't about equality. Quite the reverse. By its nature friendship is preferential: one chooses one person over another to draw closer to; an element of exclusivity is implied in the word "friend."

"Companion" is too neutral a word to be of much help in establishing what a friend is or isn't. A companion is, as it sounds, someone who happens to be in one's company. He or she may be someone on one's payroll; for example, someone an older person pays to stay with her during recovery from an illness.

Sometimes "companion" is used as a code word for a lover, which also isn't much help. A "great good friend" was the old *Time* magazine euphemism for someone a person wasn't married to but was sleeping with.

Closer to the matter are the categories of Old Friends, Out-of-Town Friends, Professional Friends, Secondary Friends, Male-Female Friends, and Ex-Friends. I won't bother to add Fair-Weather Friends, though I have a friend I call my Foul-Weather Friend, because we chiefly meet in the winter or on rainy days, since on all his other free days he is out playing golf.

Old friends include friends from one's past whom one may or may not any longer see regularly. Old friends often include friends from as far back as one's grade school or high school or college days. They might also include friends made in the military. Often these are friendships that have gone not so much sour as inactive: one of the parties to the friendship has moved to another area of the country, or perhaps once shared interests or causes or outlooks have changed, respective fortunes may have radically altered, and in the mix of all these possibilities the previous basis for the friendship has become diluted or has dissolved. A common past, or at any rate a patch of the past, is what usually unites old friends. At their best, school reunions are sustained by the feeling supplied by old friendships.

Sometimes meeting an old friend can be terribly disappointing, not to say sad, so far apart might friends have grown or so differently might they now view the world and therefore each other. Sometimes such meetings can be very sweet, especially when one still finds in an old friend, after a long lapse of time, the qualities one first liked in him or her twenty, thirty, forty, fifty and more years ago. But perhaps as often as not one finds nothing of the kind, and is left to wonder, God, what did we ever, in those distant days, find attractive in each other to begin with. Many old friendships are best left to lapse, without the drama of a final break, but simply allowed to sputter and gutter out. This becomes all the more poignant when only one party to the old friendship feels the friendship is better ended and the other wishes, hope against hope, to keep it alive. One friend may feel he has outgrown the other, to cite a common example, while the other is still entranced by the fond memories of past days and wants the friendship continued on the old basis.

Owing to American mobility — people moving about the country for work, a more pleasing environment, retirement, and much else — the category of out-of-town friend has become a larger one than perhaps at any previous time. Some friends are not merely out of town, but out of the country. One usually makes such friends through one's professional associations: scientists often meet in faraway places with colleagues from around the world; connections get made, and out of them friendships begin to form. The main — it may be a crucial — distinction between out-of-town and other friends is that the element of regularity plays a much smaller, or sometimes almost no, part in out-of-town friendships.

Good feelings can certainly stay alive with friends who live in Paris, London, Bombay, and South America, but friendship doesn't get much of a workout at such distances. The element of longing can also enter into out-of-town friendships — a longing to see the persons in question in the flesh, for which e-mails and long-distance telephone may be no substitute. I happen to have perhaps twenty friends in other cities and countries, all of whom I should like, with the wave of a magic wand, to live in the same city with me — a city, it nearly goes without saying, of perfect climate and rich cultural amenities, one agreeable to us all. Of course, it is also possible that if these fine out-of-town friendships were put to the test of reasonable regularity (a meeting every month or so), things might fall apart — presence, to reverse the old cliché, making the heart grow colder.

Not long ago I had the experience of regaining an old friend from grammar school. Back then he was the boy, so quick of mind was he, who convinced me that I had no future in mathematics. Then, in seventh grade, at the age of thirteen, he and his family moved to northern California. We had lost touch for a mere forty years when one day he sent me an e-mail, occasioned by something I had written, asking if I was the same kid with whom he had gone to Daniel Boone School in Chicago. We exchanged more e-mails, learning that, as we had common interests in those early days, we now had vastly changed but once again common interests today: sports and girls then; literature, philosophy, and art now; and an interest in baseball, then as now. When he came to Chicago a couple of years ago, so easily did we regain our former good feeling for each other, the friendship immediately rekindled. An old and lost friend, now regained, has become an out-of-town friend — I'd rather have him in town, yet reuniting with him has still been very fine.

Aristotle, in the *Nichomachean Ethics*, talks about friendships based on pleasure and friendships based on utility, neither of which, he believed, qualified as friendship of the highest order. When the pleasure was gone, when the usefulness had run its course, the friendship was finished. Yet surely everyone has had, and still has, friendships begun in the most strict utility —where one person might even have been paid to render a service to the other— that happily developed into richer friendships. Why shouldn't some of one's closest friends also be friends made in the line of work? Not for nothing are many physicians most friendly with fellow physicians, painters with painters, accountants with accountants, poets with poets.

Secondary friendships are those in which one realizes that one isn't one of the main players in the relationship, or might not have been befriended at all if another relationship hadn't first been in place. A secondary friendship is one entered into as the friend of a friend, or as the relation of a relation of a friend. One's wife, say, is dear friends with another woman, who suggests that you go out to dinner as a foursome, putting you in a friendly relationship with your wife's friend and your wife's friend's husband, whom you may or may not like. I have a friend who is in precisely such a relation in which he likes his wife's friend but strongly dislikes his wife's friend's husband, with whom he has been faking friendliness for decades. He is too good a husband, and too gentle a man, to complain; he grins and (barely) bears it.

Another category is that of specialized friendships. Specialized friends are those whom one sees only during a particular activity—tennis, golf, bridge, poker, pottery, yoga, bowling— and has no real connection with outside the specific activity. Sometimes, of course, one can first meet someone through this activity and the friendship can branch out and deepen, no longer requiring the game or craft or hobby or interest in question to keep it going. But more often, once one or the other party quits the activity, the friendship is done too.

Friendships can also be divided among those people who are older or younger or contemporary with oneself. The standard friendships — if any such thing as a standard can be said to exist in friendship — are probably those among contemporaries, who figure to have so much more in the way of common background and interests and to be at the same stage in life, which bring similar problems and pleasures and hence many more things to talk about.

My dearest friend — described in Chapter Three — was twenty-seven years older than I, though we met when I was already in my mid-thirties and he in his early sixties. But I have also had much older friends who had less experience of the world than I, and so the difference in age seemed to be wiped out, and we became equals; and in some instances, it became apparent that I, though younger, was the far more worldly person in the relationship, again wiping out age as a factor of any importance.

As one grows older, a relatively small difference in age — four years in adolescence, say, or ten or twelve in early adulthood — once providing an unpassable obstacle to friendship, seems to matter less and less and then not to matter at all. And in dead-center middle age — fifty, say — one can sometimes feel more comfortable with someone in his late seventies or early eighties than with someone in his late twenties or early thirties. Unless one is committed to the notion that the world was a good place only when one was young, which will age a person faster than any other way I know, age differences seem to count for less as one advances into late middle and early old age, and so the possibilities for friendships correspondingly widen.

And yet there remains something to the obvious fact that one's closest friends are likely to be drawn, at least for many years, from among one's contemporaries. In this wise, I have heard it said that, once one reaches eighty, everyone you meet who is eighty or beyond is not merely a contemporary but automatically a friend, though I rather doubt it. A man or woman who was a creep at forty is unlikely to improve at eighty-five.

When I was a university teacher, I of course encountered a regular supply of younger men and women, a small number of whom attracted me by their intelligence, seriousness, passion, and high spirits. We became friendly, and, as they grew older, we became actual friends, though for some there remains a barrier that, decades later, they find difficult to jump. (Two of these former students, a man now in his thirties and a woman in her forties, even today cannot bring themselves to call me by my first name, and continue to address me as Mr. Epstein.) I've met other younger men and women through my writing: they wrote to me, or we met at a public function, we stayed in touch, friendship developed. When I can, I enjoy helping bring them on in their careers, just as a few older writers helped bring me on. I hope I am never condescending to them. I would like to say that they make me feel younger; in fact, they do not. What I chiefly feel toward them is the slight protectiveness of an older friend for a younger, which is of course the true nature of our relationship. Just now we are not equals; but one day, doubtless, things will be reversed, and if I live long enough, some among them may end up feeling protective of me.

Perhaps it ought to be added that the old (or older) are pleased to the have the friendship of the young (or younger), which makes the older feel less out of the whirl of things. For many of the young — I know I felt this when younger than I now am — friendships with older men and women buck one up, making one feel that if people with long records of accomplishment behind them thought well of one, perhaps one is the person of high quality one has always, deep down, known oneself to be.

The ideal friendship, from Cicero to Montaigne, is generally posited as one between equals. Ideal it may be, but reality doesn't seem to leave much room to accommodate even near-perfect equality in friendships. Old friends who started out equal often enough find that the twists of life — good fortune, wretched luck, illness — put one or another of them well ahead, at least as the world measures the race, though friendship is best viewed outside all competition. Good character may be required for the friend who has had the better run to remain loyal to his friend, now that they are separated by money, achievement, prestige; poor character will allow him happily to desert his friend without much afterthought. Character is also required, along with the suppression of envy, for the less fortunate of the two friends not to hold his old friend's success against him. One thinks here of Gore Vidal's mean but not entirely truthless aphorism: "Whenever a friend succeeds, a little something in me dies." Francis Bacon, on this point, claims that "there is little friendship in the world, and least of all that between equals." I take Bacon's point to be that equality between people is chiefly a spur to rivalry, which can be death on friendship. And Balzac, with that worldly cynicism one comes to expect (and enjoy) in him, backs up Bacon by remarking that "nothing so fortifies a friendship as the belief on the part of one friend that he is superior to the other."

Other friendships start out unequal and remain so, equality never at any time having anything essential to do with the friendship. One may also befriend someone for qualities that are not obvious, or even knowable, until put to the test: loyalty, generosity, kindness, a good heart. Perhaps the person who has these qualities is always the one who holds an edge over the friend who is merely brilliant, attractive, or rich. Inequality, like beauty, may be only in the eye of the beholder.

Here is the place to remark again — I have already done so in my Foreword — that I do not believe either that most men cannot be close friends without a strong homoerotic element admixed, or that a man and woman cannot be friends without their not-so-secretly wishing to leap into bed with each other. Such notions are part of the rich heritage of Freudianism, whose main ideas — the Oedipus complex, the dominance of the sexual element in everyday life, the ease with which human beings repress the painful in their lives, that one's own pathetic ego must at all costs be defended — have now been plowed under by scientific evidence and covered over by common sense.

Friendships between men and women that exclude sex have become a more frequent feature of contemporary life. In my own experience, friendships between men and women can provide things that friendships between men do not. For one thing, the element of rivalrousness, sometimes present when with members of one's own sex, tends to disappear when with a member of the opposite sex on whom one has no romantic designs. For another, women, or a great many women I have known, seem more receptive to ironic and obliquely ironic points in conversation. A man can let his guard down a bit with friends who are women in a way that he is perhaps less likely to do with male friends. I can more easily imagine telling a woman that I think that clothes, far from being trivial, can be amusing or witty, and that the right clothes can on occasion make a person, man or woman, feel better than coming into possession of three fresh religious insights. Women (at least some women) are made less nervous about taking up a wider range of subjects than are men (at least most men).

In modern times there have been innumerable instances of women finding themselves greatly at ease with, in fact preferring above all others, the friendship of homosexual men. They often find such men witty, attentive to style and to the domestic arts and to the details of quotidian life in a way that heterosexual men are usually not. Gay men, too, give off the air of being socially, sometimes artistically, if not avant-garde then au courant. And for women concerned, not to say worried, about such things, homosexual men provide the additional bonus of posing no sexual threat. Homosexual men, for their part, gain from such friendships the pleasures of the purely feminine point of view, relief from the masculine pose, and entrée into a larger world than exclusively male homosexual life allows. These are of course bold — and some of them possibly already outdated — generalizations, so all exceptions to them are admitted.

The saddest category is that of ex-friends. Behind most broken friendships is a story of insensitivity, decisive sins of omission or commission, the outrages of fortune — the reasons for friendships breaking up are as manifold as those for their beginning.

Other kinds and permutations of friendship may be found, lots of them. At different times in one's life, one seeks out different sorts of friendships. Paul Valéry said that a man "has as many friends as he has personalities within him." In youth, friendships can be particularly intense. One of the consequences of marrying is that the nature of one's earlier friendships often change, though perhaps this is more true for men than for women. The degree to which one is absorbed by one's life's work will also alter the nature and number of one's friendships. The longer one lives, the fewer one's friends figure to be, and one of the sadnesses of living into one's nineties is that usually all one's friends have departed, leaving one feeling alone on the planet. No one will be surprised to learn that studies have suggested that having friends tends to lengthen the life of the elderly by, among other things, extending their interests and getting them out of themselves. Something to it, no doubt, but then one remembers some years ago other studies that claimed that the lives of the very elderly are also enriched and lengthened by having a pet to care for, which may or may not be true. As for the status of friendship in the afterlife, all such studies, and this book along with them, remain resolutely silent.

# 2

❖

# A Charming Gift for
# False Intimacy

FRIEND, AS WE HAVE SEEN, is one of those words on whose exact meaning not even dictionaries are very helpful. Friend: an attachment based on affection or esteem; a favored companion, one joined to another in mutual benevolence and intimacy; the antonym of an enemy. Having said that, one hasn't really said all that much. The difficulty is that the complications inherent in what is represented by the word "friend" aren't ever easily or quickly or efficiently formulated. The *Concise Oxford English Dictionary* definition isn't bad — "One joined to another in intimacy and mutual benevolence independently of sexual or family love" — though it leaves out a lot, including the possibility of friendship between lovers, on the one hand, and people who are not by nature given to the least intimacy, on the other. So much a matter of gradation, "friend" is a word whose meaning has to be established by comparisons, by sifting shades of difference, turned over and teased out, and after all that what one comes up with might still not feel altogether right and precise.

In Books VIII and IX of the *Nichomachean Ethics*, Aristotle, who could chop logic finer than a three-star chef can chop a Bessarabian truffle, sets out the kinds and categories of friendships as only he, most impressively comprehensive and analytical of philosophers, could do. Yet even Aristotle, great precisian though he was, could not come close to exhausting all cases, as the philosophers like to say, on the endlessly subtle subject of friends and friendship.

Wisdom inheres in Aristotle's coolly analytical sentences. He takes the wide view, which gives sweep to his outlook, and considers things from an elevated height of generality, which adds a touch of grandeur to the proceedings. "For without friends," he writes in his first paragraph on the subject, "no one would choose to live, though he had all other goods." We do not know whether Aristotle had a dear friend or what kind of friend he himself was. That he would have been an excellent friend seems likely, for no one was more thoughtful than he of what was entailed in the relation of friend to friend.

Aristotle first refers to those friendships where the main element is pleasure, or simple delight in the company of another: "the friendships of young people seem to aim at pleasure," he writes, and it is true that, when young, one tends to bounce easily in and out of friendships, looking to friends for little more than shared delight. Aristotle next considers friendships based on utility, or usefulness of each friend to the other, which takes in, at a minimum, commercial and professional and political friendships. (Tocqueville, in this connection, remarks that in politics "[shared] hatred is almost always the basis for friendship.") But friendship based on utility, according to Aristotle, is often neither of great intensity nor of noble character, for "those who are friends for the sake of utility part when the advantage is at an end."

On the relation of distance to friendship, Aristotle finds that true friendship requires that friends live close together. (My category of out-of-town friend, from the previous chapter, might present a complication to him, though of course Aristotle knew not of long-distance telephone and e-mail.) He takes up inequality in friendships, asking how much inequality a friendship can endure.

Aristotle asserts that "neither older nor sour people make friends easily"; that "goodwill is not identical to friendship"; that there are times when it makes sense to break off friendships; that "a man does not seem to have the same duties to a friend, a stranger, a comrade, and a schoolfellow"; that friends are helpful in both good times and bad; and much else. He also allows that a high degree of perfection is possible in a friendship between husband and wife, though friendship for him (as for me) is asexual in nature. On some of these points he lingers for a paragraph or so; others he merely asserts and moves on. His thoughts provide a fine outline of the subject.

But what emerges above all from Aristotle's always trenchant lucubrations is that friendship, true friendship, requires good character — in its ideal state, it calls for a selflessness that for Aristotle requires no less than nobility of character. One has to be good in oneself to qualify as a true friend, which also means one must love oneself. Which at first sounds like psychobabble reinforcing vanity, but isn't, since at the heart of genuine friendship is the golden rule (a term unavailable to Aristotle), but the golden rule practiced at the highest power, for what would be the point of treating one's friend as one does oneself if one doesn't love oneself to begin with? Perfect friendship, for Aristotle, is "the friendship of men who are good, and alike in virtue; for these wish well alike to each other *qua* good, and they are good in themselves."

To love oneself — not merely to be egotistical or to have a well-developed sense of *amour-propre* — one must, in Aristotelian terms, be genuinely worth loving. And to do that, one must have lived well: must be able to look back with reasonable happiness upon one's past, enjoy the activity of one's present, and go fearlessly on into the future. Aristotle doesn't quite say it — perhaps he does not need to — but one must be very smart about one's choice of friends and the nature of one's friendships, for, he writes, "most differences arise between friends when they are not friends in the spirit in which they think they are." At the heart of friendship for Aristotle is the love of a friend's character or of his moral virtue.

Various people have attempted to refute Aristotle's notions about friendship, and one can find many holes in them, especially in his view of a good friend being only as good as one is oneself. If one is morally superior, after all, then perhaps that is all the more reason to dispense one's good influence to people of lesser moral acuity. And if one has moral defects, why not attempt to find morally superior friends to bring oneself up to moral snuff? "To one who can do it," as the philosopher Irving Singer writes, "loving a worthless man may be more rewarding than loving a paragon of virtue." Strict adherence to the Aristotelian ideal would also severely draw in the circle of one's possible friendships, for there are surely many people of moral constitution different from one's own whose friendship is not only worthy but would probably also serve to widen one's own views in a useful — yes, even a morally useful — way.

Reading Aristotle naturally makes one reflect on the state of one's own friendships and one's own qualities and propensities as a friend. I was especially struck by the passage that holds "it would seem actually impossible to be a great friend to many people . . . we must be content if we find even a few such [excellent friends]." This point in Aristotle captured my attention because it made me realize that I have long been highly promiscuous in my friendships.

My earliest memories are of living in a neighborhood with few children my age. I spent much time by myself. I can remember afternoons when I was seven or eight, tossing a pink rubber ball against the wall of our apartment, my mother having gone out on errands. I pretended that the Chicago Cubs were playing the Boston Braves, and I systematically went through the two teams' lineups, throwing the ball for each batter, working things out so that in the end the Cubs would win. I do not recall feeling especially lonely, though technically I suppose I was.

Only when our family moved, and I found myself in a neighborhood with lots of kids my age, did I discover in myself a skill for making friends. I soon learned that I was able to persuade other boys to think well of me. I did this through making plain to them that I was, in the crucial phrase of the day, "a good guy": modest, reasonably (though not offensively) bright, someone who listened carefully, who knew his place in the status hierarchy, who was in no way pushy or selfishly on the make. I found I could cultivate boys a couple of years older than I — a vast patch of time when one is in one's adolescence — and turn them into, if not friends, at least guys in my corner. I had become something of a salesman, on the road full-time with no product in my sample case other than myself.

An older boy in my geometry class named Harry Shadian is a case in point. Although I was otherwise an indifferent high school student, I somehow had a taste and knack for geometry. I enjoyed its clarity and the opportunity it provided for plugging in theorems and axioms to answer questions. Harry, who was two years older than I and a superior athlete and an amiable guy, had no aptitude whatsoever for the subject. I let him know that I was willing to help him, by lending him my homework before class, by letting him look over my shoulder and onto my paper during exams, and whatever else I could do to get him over this hurdle. He was very appreciative and made it clear to all that I was his friend and withal a very good guy. As a friend of Harry's, my status in our large high school jumped a number of points.

I did this over and over again: sometimes for the feeling of social elevation it gave — I could get into any circle I wished — sometimes for the pleasure of exercising my essentially sales-manly gift for its own sake. I did it, moreover, without making any snobbish distinctions. I just wanted everyone to consider me his friend. Without bothering to read the book, I was exercising, with aplomb, the lessons of Dale Carnegie's then immensely successful *How to Win Friends and Influence People*, except that I had no interest in influencing anyone; I simply collected friends the way other children did stamps or seashells. ("*How to Win Friends,*" wrote Frederic Raphael, in his memoir *A Spoilt Boy*, "is probably among the dozen most blandly wicked books ever written.") "He is a worthless man," says Hesiod, in *Works and Days*, "who makes now one and now another his friend." If this were a stage and not a page, I should here have to take a bow.

As part of my prowess at making lots of friends, I had at my command a small gift for implying an intimacy that often wasn't really there. I have it still, and it sometimes gets me into difficulty, making people think I have a stronger feeling for them than in fact I do. This also, naturally enough, makes them feel that I am prepared to put myself out for them — do them favors, use such power as I have to further their causes or careers, listen at some length to their troubles — more than I truly am. I have learned to curb this too easy intimacy, but not always, I fear, sufficiently. Like other bad habits, it is not so easily shaken off.

Four or five years ago, at a gym where I used to work out, I met a serious and winning man, Charles was his name, then in his early eighties, though he seemed much younger, with whom I struck up a conversation. I told him a joke; he told me one in exchange. We were both Jewish. He was of the generation of my parents. While working rowing machines next to each other, we began to strike up regular conversations about sports, politics, whatever was in the news. He one day told me that, on the very day of his retirement from work as a cardboard-box salesman, he returned home to find his wife sitting in a chair, dead of coronary arrest. She had been a mathematics student at the University of Michigan and a science editor at *Encyclopaedia Britannica,* and was in every way the center of his life. On the same day, he said, he had left his job and lost his best friend.

He would often lapse into talking about the past, though always prefacing doing so with an apology. ("I hate to go back into the past, but . . .") He had a married son living in a nearby suburb, and granddaughters who had some of his wife's talent for science, one going to medical school, the other doing graduate study in biochemistry. A strong aura of loneliness clung to him. He was a decent man and an honorable one: when he talked politics, I always had the sense that he did so in the most admirably nonpartisan way, having the good of the country in mind. He didn't think much of Bill Clinton, for example, but deplored the way he was being hounded by the press during the year of his sex scandal: it wasn't good for the presidency, Charles felt, and hence not good for the country either.

I liked Charles a lot, and I believe he liked me. The time had come to push the relationship a bit further, changing it from pleasant acquaintanceship to friendship. All that would have been required was for me to invite him to lunch. Somehow the ball was in my court; that is, it was up to me, not him, to do so.

And with some forethought — and now some regret, too — I decided not to do anything about it. Not long after, I stopped going to this gym and lost all touch with Charles. A few years afterward I heard that, at eighty-four, he had died.

Why had I deliberately closed my heart to him, or at least to the prospect of deepening the possibilities of friendship with him? In part it was because I felt him a touch too needy; his loneliness was palpable. Would an occasional lunch really be enough? Would we soon regularize things and meet for lunch every few weeks and then, say, every Thursday? In larger part, I felt my roster of friends and acquaintances — owing to my own undiminished talent for acquiring friends — was altogether too large as it stood. I was already seeing more people — for lunches, coffees, dinners with them and their wives and husbands — than I really liked. But to my mild fraudulence was added a deep social cowardice — an inability to break things off with people who were of only peripheral interest to me. I sometimes felt I was the perfect customer for a much-needed but never produced Hallmark card that would read "We've been friends for a very long time," followed on the inside by "What do you say we stop?"

I write this with genuine trepidation, lest I become like that man whom Oscar Wilde described as having "no enemies, but he is intensely disliked by his friends." I fear that many of the people who think themselves my friends will wonder if they are among those to whom I wish to send that card. Some few are, though most are not. The problem isn't really with them but with me. I seem, in the realm of friendship, to be the equivalent, in the realm of sex, of that too fast high school girl who finds herself in the back of a Chevy, staring up at her saddle shoes and asking herself how she got here, *again.*

At the same time that I find myself overwhelmed by friends, I often find that my heart all too regularly goes out to people. I might bump into someone I haven't seen for three or four months and, in the *Gemütlichkeit* of the moment, suggest that we meet for lunch, coffee, dinner. There is not the least jot of falsity in my invitation, though there might be real regret when the time comes around for that lunch, coffee, or dinner meeting to take place. Once again there I am, on my back, studying the (now purplish) veins on my ankles in the air.

The best possible face could be put on this by saying that I am by nature a friendly person. I suppose I am, and have never seen any reason to be otherwise. Yet everywhere making friends on the one hand, I often find myself, on the other hand, grudgingly resentful of the obligations, which begin to feel more like burdens, of friendship.

Is the answer to be found in carefully delimiting the number of one's friends? Is there a perfect number of friends beyond which one is, in effect, asking not for trouble but for unnecessary complications in one's life? Aristotle sets a rough golden mean on this matter, suggesting that the number of friends a person should have is "as many as are sufficient for living together," though he does not specify a number. Plutarch somewhere says that the correct number of friends is seven. But to be specific here is to ignore the differing calibrations of friend and friendship, the varying closeness and distance of particular friendships.

An acquaintance, as I have noted in the previous chapter, is someone with whom one makes no future plans for meeting; one's relationships with acquaintances have no continuity. Less responsibility — actually no responsibility — is entailed. The element of permanence isn't a factor. "Should auld acquaintance be forgot?" Robert Burns famously asked. My answer is, why the hell not? In fact, it frequently is, for years at a time; and it turns out to be not such a bad thing. Behind most acquaintanceships is the decision, on the part of one or both parties, not to draw closer.

I was not long ago on a tour of Mitteleuropa, sponsored by a classical music station in Chicago, with thirty-five other music-minded tourists. For ten days we shared meals, attended the same concerts, ballets, and operas, rode the same buses. I found most of these people quite agreeable, with a few others I felt an easy rapport, and with one couple I believe a genuine friendship was possible. Yet on returning to the United States, I have since seen, by running into them in a supermarket, only the couple I just mentioned; nor do I long to see the others, though

I liked most of them well enough. One nice woman among them organizes annual reunions for the group, which I choose not to attend. Acquaintances they were, acquaintances they shall remain. I would only add that, since none has attempted to be in touch with me, all these people must have felt something of the same about me, which is fair enough.

Friendship speaks to a hunger to renew the pleasure of meeting. It suggests that two people haven't exhausted the delight they take in each other. Something about this person attracts me, one says upon meeting someone who is a candidate for friendship; I want to see more of him or her. We share interests, humor, background, chemistry of one kind or another. We have, one senses, things to give to each other that will enlarge and enrich both our lives.

This sense of connection that makes for friendship runs deeper in some instances than it does in others. Some years ago, I wrote an essay in which I compared my own friendships with the seating plan in a stadium, with my closest friends seated in the box seats, less close friends in the grandstand, and business associates and acquaintances in the bleachers. One could as easily change the sports metaphor from a baseball to a football field and arrange the seats of friends from dab on the fifty-yard line to high up in the end zone.

In that same essay, written twenty years ago, I declared that I had seven close friends. Two of these friends have since died; another, through not seeing him, has been removed to the grandstand; and one, without becoming anything resembling an enemy, has been permanently lost through argument. Another friend, acquired since that essay, has risen and now occupies a box seat. Still another, who started off as a neighbor, has over the years become a box-seat friend. Of these now only five close friends, no common denominator of interest exists. They vary wildly in financial fortunes, kinds of work they do, cultural interests. All have a more than decent sense of humor, with an appreciation for irony as a much-favored mode of conveying it. I do not let myself entirely loose with any one of them, but instead have different areas of reticence with each. With two among them I go back to grade and high school, where we were also close friends. Three of the five live in the same city I do, and one of these I see more than the other two. We are all past sixty, and roughly contemporaries.

My own politics and those of these friends are not congruent; in at least one case they are distinctly different. Nor am I certain of their belief in God (but, then, I am not all that confident of my own). Holding the same political or religious views isn't central to my friendships with these men. With all of them I feel I can speak with a high quotient of candor on just about any subject, even if I do not usually avail myself of the opportunity to do so. We can all also tell one another when we think the other is wrong, or possibly full of crap, without the danger of the friendship breaking down. In the company of any of them, very little front need be maintained: I can be pretty much myself with them and assume they feel they can be likewise with me.

As close as I feel to these men, my relationship with none of them can be described as in any way therapeutic — including with the one of them who is a practicing psychiatrist. I share with them a core of beliefs that might go by the name of manly stoicism. We prefer to think that we have strong radar for spotting BS. Each of us can read the other's signals. We agree on what is funny in the world. We have also agreed, tacitly, to overlook one another's flaws. We do not bitch, whine, or cry in one another's presence.

Where friendship becomes complicated is in the range of grandstand friends, of whom, though I have not made a careful count, I may have forty or fifty, maybe more. Part of the reason for this large number is that I live in the city in which I grew up, and regularly run into people whose friendships I cultivated when young. Through my writing I've acquired a number of friends in other American cities, and a few good friends in England, and one who now lives in Israel. Many of my friendships with people living in other cities seem to me full of a promise that, as they and I grow older, will probably never come to fruition. Such is my good feeling about them that, but for the want of proximity, several, I suspect, could easily become box-seat or fifty-yard-line friends. And yet if all of them lived in

Chicago, I might get no work done whatsoever, but go under, drowned in waves of friendship.

Another category of friends is composed of twenty or so former students I felt a special pull toward, of the few thousand students I must have taught during thirty years at Northwestern University. Some among them are now in their forties and early fifties. While in the classroom, I ignited a spark in them, and they in me, and we have stayed in touch over the years. Inequality slightly marks these friendships, because I am older by at least fifteen years than all of them and I was once in a position of authority over them. They benefited, I believe, from my taking their intellectual and artistic aspirations seriously. I benefited, in vaguer but still genuine ways, from their regard. But at one point or another, I felt for them something of the love—nonerotic division—that Plato cites as part of the true relation between teacher and student.

In all these good but secondary friendships what is missing is an element of regularity. When I see these men and women in my grandstand seats, I enjoy myself greatly in their company and yet know that a long while may pass before we are in any sort of contact again—in some cases it could be years. Nothing wrong with this; in fact, from a certain point of view it's a relief: to attempt to maintain so many friendships on a regular basis would turn me into a professional friend. My feeling for all these people—which of course I hope is reciprocated—is real, but for one reason or another neither party feels the need to sustain it through regularized meetings. Still, good friends we are nonetheless.

Which reminds me that I have come this far without attempting a definition of my own of a friend. The best I can provide at this point is rather a baggy-pants one for friendship generally: friendship is affection, variously based on common interests, a common past, common values, and, alas, sometimes common enemies, in each case leading to delight and contentment in one another's company. As for what constitutes the basis for friendship, this, too, can be wildly various. In his autobiographical Orchid Trilogy, the English author Jocelyn Brooke writes of a good friend of his early manhood that "we were unable to take each other or (when we were together) our respective selves *au grand sérieux*. It is, I suppose, as good a foundation for friendship as any other; better, perhaps, than most." The obliquity of that definition — a friend is someone one likes a great deal without having to take altogether seriously — is oddly appealing.

The hunt for synonyms for the word "friend" provides further fodder for definition, but it, too, finally isn't all that helpful. Other self, soul mate, confidant, ally, chum, crony, buddy, alter ego, *copain* — a friend can be all of these things, or a combination of a few of them, and also none of them. Perhaps the best way to define a friend, at least for now, is not through formulating a precise definition but through attempting to understand the obligations inherent in the relationship between people who wish to think of themselves as friends. Paradoxical as it may seem, without obligations — sometimes damn irritating ones — there may be no real basis for friendship.

# 3

❖

# *Best Friends*

WHEN ONE THINKS of friendship, one's mind soon turns to that friend of all friends, the best friend. From David and Jonathan in the Old Testament to Huckleberry Finn and Jim in literature to Butch and Sundance in the movies, the relationship of best friends is rich and ripe and fruitful in too many ways to count. A best friend is that person who gives you the most delight, support, and comfort, often in those realms where family cannot help. A best friend is perhaps the only person to whom you can complain about the difficulties presented by your family. In the ideal version — more precisely, in the idealized version — a best friend is someone with whom you can joke freely, be serious comfortably, be open easily, never worrying about giving offense. A best friend is, as the philosopher George Santayana once put it, the person with whom you "can be most human," which is another way of saying, be most yourself.

A best friend is frequently taken to be like a brother or sister, possibly to a higher power — somehow, again ideally, even better. An old boyhood rite, copied from the cowboy movies of the 1940s, had two young boys cut their fingers and each rub his cut finger with that of his friend, thus establishing them as blood brothers. A best friend is in some ways a more sacred relation than any other, for it is freely chosen (unlike a family relationship) and the commitment, entered into voluntarily, is somehow felt to be deeper. Anyone who has had a best friend will know the exhilarating feeling of closeness and partnership it yields; anyone who has never had such a friend has missed out on one of life's great pleasures.

And yet might the notion of best friends be overidealized? Does the intensity of such a friendship put too much pressure on both parties to the friendship? Such a friendship assumes, if not an equality of status, an equality of feeling, one friend for the other, and this entails a delicate balance that can be easily overturned, if not betrayed, by the least tincture of advantage, envy, or absence of perfect reciprocity. William Maxwell's novel *The Folded Leaf* provides an account of two boys whose close friendship sours and then withers when they go off to college and the appeal of the more physically gifted of the two is superseded by the greater spiritual quality of the other.

Michel de Montaigne (1533–1592) claimed a sublime best friendship with Étienne de La Boétie (1530–1563). Montaigne was — or one day would be — the famous author of the *Essais* and the man who first brought the "I," or first-person singular, into literature. He was the Homer and the Shakespeare of the personal essay, a form he invented. His essay "On Friendship" has remained one of the key documents on the relations among friends.

The friendship between La Boétie and Montaigne lasted four years. La Boétie died at thirty, and Montaigne would go on to live another twenty-nine years. Montaigne claimed that he turned to writing essays because, with his dear friend dead, he had no one to whom he could reveal himself with the same intimacy that he was able to do with Étienne. "What we ordinarily call friends and friendships are nothing but acquaintanceships and familiarities formed by some chance or convenience, by means of which our souls are bound to each other," Montaigne wrote. "In the friendship I speak of [that with La Boétie], our souls mingle and blend with each other so completely that they efface the seam that joined them, and cannot find it again. If you press me to tell you why I loved him, I feel that this cannot be expressed, except by answering: Because it was he, because it was I."

Montaigne and La Boétie likely met in 1559, when both were members of the Bordeaux legislative assembly. They knew of each other by reputation. The note of mutual high regard was struck at their first meeting. Étienne was two and a half years older than Michel, married (as Michel at the time was not), and of a more conservative cast of mind. Donald Frame, Montaigne's biographer and translator, believes that La Boétie, being the more experienced man, was also the leader, or "mentor," a now overused word, in the relationship. They called each other brother. La Boétie wrote that "there is no reason to fear that our descendants, if only the fates permit, will begrudge placing our names among those of famous friends." And so, because of the power of Montaigne's essay, they have been placed, imperishably.

On his deathbed, La Boétie willed Montaigne his library, and Montaigne was with him at his bedside as he departed the world. After La Boétie's death, Montaigne had inscribed on the walls of the tower that was his study: "[To the shades of Étienne de La Boétie], the tenderest, sweetest, and closest companion, than whom our age has seen no one better, more learned, more charming, or indeed more perfect . . ."

In his essay, Montaigne uses his friendship with La Boétie to launch an interesting guide to the different kinds of friendships, their utility and their limitations. As was his habit, he quotes from the classical authors to back up his points. He takes up the responsibilities of fathers to sons and sons to fathers, and remarks that these are limited by the "fear of begetting an unbecoming intimacy," a fear that no longer, it is true, exists among us in the twenty-first century, but was real enough in Montaigne's day. Besides, the relationship between parents and children is bound by a sense of obligation, each to the other, and hasn't the quality of disinterest, of impartial love for its own sake, that deep friendship, in Montaigne's sense of it, requires.

The friendships between siblings — brother and brother, sister and sister, brother and sister — suffer under some of the same limitations and constraints. But even if they didn't, there is, Montaigne contends, no reason why two children born of the same parents should have all that much in common, for they can be utterly different in their temperaments, interests, points of view. He cites Plutarch quoting a man, in response to being pressed to reconcile with his brother, remarking: "He matters no more to me for coming out of the same hole."

Nor did relationships between men and women qualify for the kind of heightened friendship Montaigne had had with La Boétie. "You cannot compare with friendship the passion men feel for women, even though it is born of our own choice, nor can you put them in the same category." The problem here, in Montaigne's view, was sex, which always raised, one shouldn't say its ugly, but at least its insistent, head. Sexual love, he believed, has a madness to it that is in contradiction to the love of friends, which has a "general universal warmth, temperate moreover and smooth, a warmth which is constant and at rest, all gentleness and evenness, having nothing sharp nor keen" about it.

In our own day, the question of whether great friendships between men and women can exist untouched by sexual feeling is in the flux of continuing controversy, but not for Montaigne, who didn't believe that the kind of friendship he most admired — and shared exclusively with Étienne de La Boétie — was possible even in marriage. The notion of one's wife being one's best friend is one he rejected, believing marriage to be "a bargain struck for other purposes: within it you soon have to unsnarl hundreds of extraneous tangled ends, which are enough to break the thread of a living passion and to trouble its course, whereas in friendship there is no traffic or commerce but with itself." Montaigne's own marriage, there is reason to believe, was not unrelievedly felicitous. In the spirit of his time, he rarely gave women the benefit of any doubt, and he didn't believe that women were near capable of the selfless friendship he claimed to have known with La Boétie.

Montaigne went against his beloved ancient Greeks in rejecting the idea of pederasty, the love between an older man and a boy, as a form of ideal friendship. He called pederasty "rightly abhorrent to our manners," and disqualified it further because it tended to be "simply based on physical beauty." He added that "since as they practiced [pederasty], it required a great disparity of age and divergence of favors between the lovers, it did not correspond either to that perfect union and congruity which we are seeking here." The element of equality, however rough, was missing — and in friendship equality, for Montaigne, was fundamental. Friendship for him was "a kind of love more equable and more equitable," which he caps with a quotation from Cicero: "Such only are to be considered friendships in which characters have been confirmed and strengthened with age."

The remainder of the essay is a paean to La Boétie and their friendship. All differences and divisions, Montaigne claims, were washed away in their friendship; duty, gratitude, and the rest simply didn't exist between them. They could neither lend nor give each other anything, for what one owned was felt to be in the possession of the other. "For the perfect friendship that I am talking about is indivisible: each gives himself so entirely to his friend that he has nothing left to share with another . . . The unique, highest friendship loosens all other bonds."

If in reading this rhapsodic account you feel you have yourself had no friendship that comes close to equaling it, you are not to despair, for Montaigne could find no other like it, either, in his personal experience or in his vast reading: "For the very writings which Antiquity have left us on the subject seem weak to me compared to what I feel."

For a writer a good part of whose charm was his ability to render specific detail — read him, for instance, on the pain of his kidney stones — Montaigne leaves his prose portrait of Étienne de La Boétie rather vaporous and wraith-like, as is of course perfection itself. Why did Montaigne fail to fill in his picture of this dearest of all friends with enlivening detail? Why is there so disappointing a paucity of useful anecdotes, incidents, examples set before us to bring the glory of this most beautiful of friendships to life?

Might it be that Montaigne, when he came to write about this friendship, which was at least seven years after La Boétie's death, remembered only the glow and not the fire of his great bond? "His was indeed an ample soul, beautiful from every point of view, a soul of the Ancient mould which would have brought forth great achievements if his fate had so allowed." Isn't it possible, in other words, that Montaigne exaggerated, idealized, maybe fantasized things a bit? One cannot with certitude say. All one can do is to run a reality check of Montaigne against one's own friendships, in the hope of discovering anything like the same qualities in them as he found in his friendship with Étienne.

Over a longish life, I have had several best friends. When I was a boy, I took on and scraped off best friends the way a careful boat owner does barnacles. I seemed to have a fresh best friend every summer, and sometimes I would have different best friends for different activities. I might have a best friend at grammar school and another best friend with whom to ditch Hebrew school, which I did a fair amount. There was a boy who qualified as my best friend during the two or three years, between thirteen and sixteen, when I was passionate about tennis. Sitting on the bench as a sub on my high school's frosh-soph basketball team, I had a best friend — for four months — with whom I had in common the grievance of each of us thinking himself better than many of those who got into games ahead of us: ours was a bitching friendship, for bitching was what we mostly did together.

Some of these friendships broke up over trivial (though it didn't seem so at the time) arguments. Some merely lapsed. Most were, with time, demoted to friendships of lesser intensity. I had two friends whom for a very long while I thought of as, collectively, my best friend; and today, nearly sixty years later, they are still among my "best" friends, though we can go for weeks, sometimes months, without seeing one another. When I was a boy, a best friend was someone I could pal around with in nearly total comfort, around whom I could drop much of my usual reticence, and count on just about completely. But, please note, my previous sentence bristles with qualifiers: nearly, much of, just about. I have never had a friend with whom these qualifications didn't apply, and in the time left to me I do not expect to have such a friend.

·   ·   ·

In the years between those of the grammar school playground and late middle age, I made contact with a large number of new friends. But while I was married (twice), male companionship, though still important to me, played a somewhat diminished part in my life. The truth is that from the time I was young, I had a respectable skill at making, if not necessarily for maintaining, new friends. No one existed, I thought, whom, with the aid of my essentially salesmanly skills, I couldn't befriend. I even took a certain perverse pride in making friends with people from backgrounds as different from mine as was possible within the borders of the same country. In the army, when I was in basic training at Fort Leonard Wood, the man who slept in the bunk above mine was a Christian Scientist named Chester Cook, from a small town in Kansas. He was balding, pinkish, used no profanity, was mild-mannered, good-hearted, decent in every regard. I liked him straightaway, and he soon came to like me. I led him to believe that, despite all our differences in background, we might become close friends — in the context of the army, at any rate, something resembling best friends. But I also soon found myself deserting him in small ways, going off with more lively guys in our platoon, spending less and less time with him as the weeks of training progressed, until what had begun as a friendship faded into little more than an acquaintanceship. When we separately went off to our next posting, we did not bother to pretend that we would stay in touch, with the hope of meeting again one day. Betrayal is what it was — I betrayed him, not in any way him me. Did I feel guilty about this? Yes, and decades later I still do.

I mention this because I sometimes think I no longer have the makings of a best friend. I am, I think, a decent listener, but not much of a confessor. I have a natural sense of reticence, at least when it comes to spilling my own beans, probably inherited from my parents, who were among the world's least therapeutic-minded people. I hold with the novelist Cesare Pavese that "one stops being a child when one realizes that telling one's troubles does not make things better."

Shortly before he died, Edward Shils, the friend who has meant more to me than any other, said, after acknowledging my telling him how important his friendship was to me, that I had been a dear friend to him, "even though we rarely spoke of things of the heart." What he meant, I think, was that we didn't share our disappointments, sorrows, griefs. And it is true; we did not. Did he, I am now left to wonder, long to do so with me?

Yet I loved him, and on all other subjects — money, friends in common, family — we spoke freely and easily. My trust in him was complete. He was twenty-seven years older than I, and more intelligent, wiser, in every way. I learned much more from him than he from me. We were, I like to think, equally generous to each other. I loved to give him things: books, mildly exotic foods, sweaters and neckties. When he died he left me two valuable sculptures and left my wife a beautiful set of English bone-china dishes, off which we dine every night, a splendid gift, not least because it causes me to remember him every day of my life.

We were of different generations. He was old enough to have lived through the Depression and served in World War II, while I knew the latter only as a child and the former only by hearsay. His worldliness was vastly greater than mine; he had taught in England for decades, lived in India, knew important intellectual figures in every country in Europe. His tone was international; mine, certainly next to his, provincial. He attempted to internationalize me, at least a little. He regularly introduced me to writers and scholars from Poland, Germany, Hungary, Italy, and England. It was one of his many gifts to me.

My first gift to him was a set of eight small porcelain Charles Dickens characters. I loved these figurines, but I felt he loved them more, which pleased me to give them to him. He didn't drive a car, and we lived twenty miles apart, but I never minded picking him up for dinner or other meetings, so exhilarating was it for me to be with him. Among his many talents was that of a high comic perspective: he could evaluate — and smash — other people's pretensions as no one else I have ever known. He could calibrate a person's strengths without neglecting his weaknesses. He made plain the rewards of intellectual passion through the example of his own life and work.

What his friendship offered me was obvious. What mine of-

fered him is less so. Ours was decidedly a friendship of un-
equals, though he had too much tact ever to underscore this in
our day-to-day relations. Perhaps it comforted him to know that
someone much younger than he knew his value. He knew that I
could pick up all the nuances of his wit, which could be extremely subtle and wildly funny. He could show his playful side
to me as perhaps to few other people. Once, when we were din-
ing at the University of Chicago faculty club, I pointed out that
every item on the menu seemed to have a place name attached
to it: spaghetti Bolognese, meatloaf Peruvian, and so on. "Yes,"
he said, "our chef has long had a fine grasp of geography. If
only the son-of-a-bitch would now acquire a cookbook."

In me he had someone with whom he could be utterly candid in his assessment of people and events. If we disagreed,
which we almost never did, it was the disagreement of people
who knew they agreed on fundamental things. We felt, or so I
believe, a genuine comfort in each other's company. He had
other friends, other people he loved, but I like to think that in
me he sensed an unqualified support of his ideas and of the way
he had chosen to live — a support behind which lay a nearly
complete understanding of his motives and his reasoning and,
finally, the meaning of his life.

I'm less than certain how to describe the nature of our
friendship. He was no father figure to me — having had a good
father, I had no need for another — he was not avuncular and
not a mentor, though I learned a vast amount from him. He was
not the older brother I never had, for our being of different generations eliminated that possibility. I found him to be intellectually heroic, but I knew him too well for him to be an unqualified
hero. What we were was dear friends, and I felt myself lucky —
blessed, really — to have been chosen by him as someone he
wished to spend a lot of time with, could to some degree confide in, and showed affection toward.

On his deathbed, Étienne de La Boétie told Montaigne: "My
brother, my friend, I assure you that I have done many things in
my life, it seems to me, with as much pain and difficulty as I do
this. And when all is said, I had been prepared for it for a very
long time and had known my lesson by heart." My friend Ed-

ward, who once described himself as a "pious agnostic," by which he meant that he greatly respected religion but could not make the leap into faith, told me that he thought he had the character to meet death unflinchingly. And, after a long bout with cancer, involving two rounds of strong chemotherapy, he did—honorably, courageously, with a serenity of the kind that philosophy is supposed to imbue in those who have learned its lessons well.

Montaigne spent the rest of his days missing La Boétie, and I have felt something of the same emotion for Edward. I often see or hear or read things that I want to tell him; sometimes I imagine—with reasonable accuracy, I think—his reactions to events, books, people. He died, my friend, when I was fifty-eight. I am sixty-seven as I write this, and I sense that this was easily the most important male friendship of my life, and that, like Montaigne's with Étienne de La Boétie, I shan't, for the remainder of my days, have another to equal it.

And yet . . . and yet can I claim perfection in my friendship of the kind that Montaigne claimed in his for La Boétie? My friendship was near perfect, but it wasn't the pure ideal that Montaigne makes his seem. I can recall moments of exasperation with my dear friend—moments recollected not in tranquility, to be sure, but in mild yet genuine guilt—when I felt he was carrying on much too long in the spirit of tirade when attacking people or institutions; usually, let me add, people or institutions richly worthy of attack. But it seemed as if, in his anger, he lost his sense of measure and hence of control. During such moments, I merely waited for him to finish, my mind turned to cruise control.

In his last years he became harder and harder of hearing, but chose not to get a hearing aid. In conversation, because of his poor hearing, I would find myself almost shouting at him. Shouting does nothing to improve intimacy or to encourage witty response. How maddening, I thought. How much of what I am saying is he hearing? I wondered. Because of this, I felt a slight futility enter our conversations, at least from my side.

Sometimes I would find him veering away from what I considered reality. He would on occasion encourage people to intellectual enterprise — finishing a doctorate, writing a book, recording in memoirs the years of their upbringing — that I thought them incapable of achieving. His standards were so high that he could write a recommendation for a former student that, because it was utterly truthful, was automatically disqualifying. He didn't seem to understand that in a university recommendation, truth isn't at all what is required; hyperbole is.

He could be rigid in his formality, unbending in his standards. He never appeared outside his home without a tie and jacket, and my guess is that he judged harshly those men who did. We used to go to the restaurant of a Chinese chef whose cooking was unsurpassed. One day I said to my friend, "You know, Edward, I think Mr. Moy would like it a lot if you would call him Ben, which would allow him to call you by your first name." He thought a moment, then answered, "I can't," and I knew the subject was forever closed.

None of these things made me love him less. But they were small imperfections that I now recall in the light of the absolutely clean slate that Montaigne accords La Boétie. Of course, I knew my dear friend for twenty-four years, whereas Montaigne knew his for a mere four. Nor do I know what imperfections — and worse — he might have found in me; hypercritical as he was, these could not have been few.

My larger point is that no friendship, contra Montaigne, is perfect. Some are fine, splendid, charmed, wondrous, but none is without flaw. Perfection in friendship just isn't on the menu. To idealize friendship, in general or in particular, is a serious error, and to require Montaigne's "perfect union and congruity" in friends is, I have come to believe, the gravest of mistakes.

# 4

❖

# *The Quickest Way to*
# *Kill Friendships*

WHEN A BOARD OF ACADEMICS was discussing the possibility of my being fired from an editorial job I then held, it was reported to me that one man on the board said, "I can never vote in favor of this, of course, because I am Joe's friend." I had always liked this man but until then had not realized the depth of my good feeling for him, chiefly because he showed in a public way how seriously he took the responsibility of friendship. I greatly admired the certitude of his simple statement — "because I am Joe's friend" — and all that it implied of the duties owed to friendship, loyalty not least among them.

Not long after, when I reported to a regular contributor to the magazine about a reviewer I had chosen for a new book of his, he wrote back to say that there was much bad feeling between him and the reviewer, who was likely to write an unfair attack on the book. I realized at that moment how I had come to think of this man as a friend, and so I wrote back to him: "Not only would I not permit an unfair attack on your book to appear in any magazine I edit, but be assured that I wouldn't even allow a fair attack."

Loyalty is certainly among the responsibilities of friendship, but to what degree? "All for one and one for all!" exclaimed D'Artagnan and the Three Musketeers in Alexander Dumas's famous novel, formulating the high ideal of loyalty among friends. Yet one wonders. One wonders if Porthos mightn't have told Athos that he thought Aramis was a bit cheap ("You'd think once, just once, he'd pick up the tab for a flagon of Bordeaux"); if Aramis ever asked Porthos whether he noticed that Athos's breath was not all it should be; if Athos told Aramis that Porthos, when you got right down to it, was damn pushy; and if, after a night's drinking, the three men tended to agree that D'Artagnan's flair was overdone and made him seem — how to say this? — just a touch light in the loafers.

All of which is to say that in friendships, as in almost every other sphere of life, vast discrepancies exist between the ideal and reality. A *New Yorker* cartoon has a man coming out of a church exclaiming, "How can I love my enemies when I don't even like my friends?" Life provides moments when, alas, one knows whereof the fellow speaks. "Thy friendship oft has made my heart to ache," wrote William Blake. "Do be my enemy — for friendship's sake."

The language available to us today to talk about friendships isn't impressively precise. We speak of "relationships," of "relating to," of "identifying" and "empathizing" with friends — all of which seems to me Play-Doh language, words that can be shaped to almost any meaning one likes. More elegant, foreign-born words — rapport, simpatico — aren't always helpful either in describing the nature of, let alone the motives for, friendship. Nor is it certain that we can invent the necessary language. So rich, so varied, so different from the ideal are friends and friendships — especially those of today — likely to be that it sometimes seems that all we can do is describe friendships one at a time, as if each is sui generis, which every one may very well be. "It is no accident," writes the English sociologist Digby Anderson, in *Losing Friends*, "that the friendship literature has few theories about friendship but is stuffed with actual stories about friends."

Why does one decide to befriend one person rather than another, at least when such friendships are made deliberately and not by accident? And so many friendships are, it would seem, made by accident, or near accident: he sat next to me in class, she took her child to the same park I took mine to, we both worked in the advertising department at Sears, and so on.

The first friendship I can recall making a clear decision about occurred when a new boy transferred to our grammar school in the seventh grade. I myself had transferred there two years earlier. Between the ages of five and ten, as I've mentioned, I hadn't many friends, and spent much time alone. I had a strong suspicion that in life's drama I had been cast as a peripheral character. When I transferred to a new school in a different neighborhood, I suddenly found myself thought a good athlete and was put in all the prime positions — shortstop, quarterback, point guard — on our playground teams. Moving in from the periphery, I was now a central character. People sought me as a friend.

When in the seventh grade this new boy arrived from a nearby school, I sensed right away that I wanted him for my friend. What was it about him that I found attractive? We had the common interests of twelve-year-old boys — sports, goofing off, an incipient taste for the nuttiness of language — but I liked above all his combination of good humor and generosity. He was intelligent and as far as possible from being a pig of egotism; he did not require the limelight or push himself forward for attention at every chance. He had a good-hearted modesty. He listened fully as much as he talked, maybe even a little more.

Soon after we became friends, I remember his asking me if I thought I could punch someone in the face. I said that I didn't think it would present a problem for me. He told me that he could never do so, that the thought actually sickened him. He wasn't cowardly, but he had a better imagination for pain — certainly for the next fellow's pain — than I. Imagination and selflessness were central to his character. He has remained my friend more than half a century later.

Other friendships came to me naturally, mainly through the classroom, for in grammar school it was rare to be close friends with anyone not in one's "room." But I consciously shied away from boys who I sensed did not qualify as friends. These were boys who were too vain, or too readily promoted themselves and their own interests — who were, in effect, in business for themselves. I had already begun to feel about them, as I still feel more strongly today, that they are not really candidates for friendship, at any rate not with me.

"A face that only a mother could love" was an expression of my mother's generation that applied to homely children, and there are people so selfish, ornery, and otherwise disagreeable that one wonders how they could have any friends at all. Yet often enough they do. One can only speculate as to why. Do they attract equally unpleasant people as friends? Or merely people who use friendship as an outlet for their masochism? Or are all the friendships of such people built on the strictly utilitarian grounds of mutual—and temporary—usefulness? We are in the midst here of another of life's manifold mysteries.

Not that some among these people are without their own odd allure. When I was younger, I myself fell for a few of them. As a high school kid, I ran for a brief spell with a boy eighteen months older than I who had astonishing freedom backed up by lots of money (owing to a newly rich and less than fully interested father) and a taste for corruption. Running around with him made life seem thrilling: lots of gambling, sexual adventures, entrée to places whose doors were usually closed to teenage boys. But the understanding here was that I was without any prospect of ever being his equal. Yet subordinating myself, for a short while, was all right—it was worth the price of glimpses of a different and exciting world that came as the dividend. But genuine friendship was not a real possibility.

Detecting who is in business solely for him- or herself can be a subtle matter. In a sense, we are all in business for ourselves. I am ready to go broke for the education or health of my grandchildren, though I would be willing to lend only a limited amount of money to even a dear friend who came to me for financial help for his children or grandchildren. Friendship often has limits that relations between parents and children do not. How far is one willing to share one's good fortune with friends? Ought one to expect friends to make at least partially good one's own failures? Probably not. But all this is far from clear, very far.

In World War II, men said of certain fellow soldiers that they

were the men they wanted with them in their foxhole. By this
they meant that these were guys whom they could count on absolutely for courage and honor; they would be there when
needed; they would never let you down; they would come
through under the worst of circumstances.

I know people whom I would want in my foxhole but whom
I do not consider close friends, or even friends at all. And I have
friends, good friends, whom I would not want anywhere near
my foxhole, because courage and loyalty under pressure aren't
things for which I would ever count on them, though they have
other excellent qualities.

When I have chosen friends — and in many cases the choice
has not been all that deliberate — they have been people who
have been honest; they have had a sense of humor, though this
quality is naturally stronger in some than in others. I don't
much care about the politics of a friend, and I have friends
across the political spectrum, but I prefer a friend whose personality is not dominated by his politics. I could not be friendly
with a closed-hearted racist or a cold (or hot) anti-Semite.
Less than shocking to report, given my squareness, which I prefer to consider merely ironic conformity, I do not have any male
friends who have ponytails or female friends with large tattoos.

One of the comforts of friends is shared references; one can
allude to certain things — historical events, song lyrics, cultural
phenomena — without having to supply either footnotes or a
glossary. Yet I cannot claim that all, or even many, of my friends
could respond to my mentioning Lord Berners or Robert de
Montesquiou, or could fill me in on the lyrics to Louis Armstrong's "I Guess I'll Get the Papers and Go Home," just as I
could not respond to their mention of things that are specialties
in their homes. But we all find things to talk about; and above
and beyond these things we have in common certain unspoken
assumptions about what is and what isn't important in life. This
makes it possible for us to laugh together. Unless you have settled morals, Virginia Woolf wrote, you can't know what to laugh
at. At this stage in life, it would be difficult for me to have anything approaching a close friendship with someone who isn't
sure what he or she ought to find amusing.

Perhaps the quickest way for me to lose interest in possible friendship with a person is for him or her to drop all reticence soon after meeting and shift directly into confessional-intimacy mode. I do intimacy well only with my wife, but even before I married I shied away from deep intimacy with friends. Francis Bacon, in his essay "Of Friendship," thought confession one of the highest functions of friendship: Bacon wrote of the great value of a true friend "to whom you may impart griefs, joys, fears, hopes, suspicions, counsels, and whatsoever lieth upon the heart to oppress, in a kind of civil shrift or confession." All this is distinctly not my idea of a good time. If I strongly felt the need for regular confession, I would consider psychoanalysis or the Catholic Church.

Nor do I often avail myself of Bacon's other main reasons for friendship: "to rehearse and work through my own thoughts and views in the mirror of another's mind, and [gain] faithful counsel on the rightness of my judgements and position in the world." I sometimes try out such ideas as I have on friends, but it is not for this that I chiefly value them. I do not ask them for financial or medical or literary advice. I pay literary agents and lawyers and doctors for such things; paying brings with it the right to be angry with or quit such people if they are wrong.

Although I talk with friends about serious things, these things are generally outside the realm of the personal. I prefer to keep my failures and disappointments to myself. Perhaps I pride myself too much on the soundness of my own judgment, but why should I trust even very good friends to know better than I whether a decision I plan to make is good or bad? Because, I suppose the standard answer is, they can sometimes view things more objectively. Yet I go on the assumption that, friends though they be, they have other things to worry about; and while, being friends, they doubtless have my welfare at heart, how can I expect them to know more about my life than I do? What I do hope from friends is that, around them, I can drop all pretensions and other protective coloring and pretty much be myself; that they can do the same around me; and together, somehow, we can make our own good music together.

One would expect the view, so therapeutic in its impulses,

that friendship is mainly about mutual confession to be of recent origin, but it is in fact of rather long standing. Ralph Waldo Emerson writes: "The scholar sits down to write, and all his years of mediation do not furnish him with one good thought or happy expression; but it is necessary to write a letter to a friend — and, forthwith, troops of gentle thoughts invest themselves, on every hand, with chosen words." Not for me they don't, or at least not usually; and my guess is that they didn't either for those people who received Emerson's sententious letters.

So much of past writing about friendship, especially when the subject is taken up in the abstract, runs from the idealized on up to the dithyrambic. Here is Emerson again, with the helium machine turned all the way up: "The moment we indulge our affections, the earth is metamorphosed; there is no winter, and no night; all tragedies, all ennuis, vanish — all duties even; nothing fills the proceeding eternity but the forms all radiant of beloved persons." Interesting to note here that Emerson himself claimed never to have such a friendship, allowing that "I have never known so high a fellowship as others." My own guess is that not many others are likely to have known it, too.

Emerson returns to earth when he writes that "a friend is a person with whom I may be sincere. Before him I may think aloud. I am arrived at last in the presence of a man so real and equal, that I may drop even those undermost garments of dissimulation, courtesy, and second thought, which men never put off, and may deal with him with the simplicity and wholeness with which one chemical meets another." To reduce the high-octane content in Emerson's language, if not entirely slip back into "those undermost garments of dissimulation": he is obviously right when he says that a greater candor is permitted among friends. Friends are often able to talk to each other in a spirit of freedom, in a happy let's-cut-the-crap atmosphere not generally permitted among nonfriends or acquaintances. And I suppose that one of the things one looks for in a friend, or when considering taking on a new friend, is the possibility of easy candor in conversation.

Yet once again I have to report that even among dear friends I am far from complete in revealing my feelings or innermost thoughts. I find that I confess to no friends and confide in very few. When I do confide, it is often about little more than what I paid for this or that, my slight disappointment in something or other not working out as I had hoped, my true opinion about a common acquaintance. Usually these modest confidences are returned.

While I have held many friends dear, I have never had one that I thought of as a confidant, certainly not on a regular basis. And I have never used a friend for regular confession. Possibly this is because, in a quiet life, I haven't had all that much interesting to confess. (Nor have I availed myself of psychotherapy, which might be viewed as secular, high-priced, and prepaid confession, with few of the genuine pleasures of friendship attached.) More likely it is because I don't wish to burden friends with such meager inner turmoil as I possess; and I like to think I wouldn't if I did have the inner turmoil in sufficient intensity to require release. All I have to confess are the standard (and boring) human miseries: little greeds, pathetic envies, the occasional feeling of being slighted at others' underestimating my charms and talents.

In a fortunate life, I have had only two serious (nonmedical) setbacks: I went through a divorce in my early thirties and I lost a son in his twenty-eighth year, when I was myself fifty-three. I wrote a book about divorce without mentioning my then ex-wife; and about the death of my son I have spoken at length to no one except my second (and final) wife. A friend who is a psychiatrist, subsequently a good friend, once asked me, in the spirit of kindness, if I cared to talk to him about it. I said no, thank you. The only one I care to talk to about it is God, though thus far He hasn't answered any of my queries on the subject.

If, then, I look to friends neither for confession nor for confiding, what then do I require of them? Frequent meetings are not required. Chekhov said of his late-life (late for him, who died at forty-four) marriage to the actress Olga Knipper that she was like the moon in his life, someone he cared a great deal about but didn't necessarily want in his sky every evening. As Chekhov said about his relations with his wife, I would say about even my dearest friends: I don't wish them in my sky every night, and I'm confident that they feel the same about me.

I also don't wish to take on any new friends who are staggering under the sadness of their lives, though I am ready to stand by old friends who have, in the all-too-efficient way life has of bringing this about, broken down in one of manifold possible ways. A little ping went off when I read, in David Cecil's life of the writer and artist Max Beerbohm, that Beerbohm sometimes "thought he preferred the company of acquaintances to that of friends. Acquaintances were too much on their good behavior openly to exhibit their weaknesses."

In my late sixties, I continue to make new friends. Those I find congenial tend to laugh a fair amount. The element of absurdity in the world is not lost on them. They are not over-impressed with their own virtue or the chances of the world perfecting itself soon. They do not lapse into unconscious self-congratulation, nor are they vain about their own or their children's or grandchildren's accomplishments. Insofar as it is possible for human beings to be, they are free of envy, major and minor snobberies, one-upmanship, rivalrousness generally. Such competitiveness as they have is properly placed in doing their work well and not dissipated on dopey competition with friends. If they are ambitious, theirs is ambition with something more behind it than sheer getting ahead.

People I consider for friends — leaving aside the question of their wishing to consider me for a friend — have a quality that I can only call *seriousness,* adding that this seriousness does not preclude great good humor, whimsy, even clownishness. Seriousness has, though, to do with recognizing, if rarely enunciating, that the human drama is about trying to determine what is and is not significant in a finite life. Seriousness has to do with attempting to make sense of one's experiences, not least one's sufferings and setbacks. Seriousness lends gravity to a man or woman, gravity that, if this not be a physical contradiction, does not weigh them down.

In his early forties, the novelist Evelyn Waugh claimed that he made one new friend every year and lost two. (Given Waugh's style of calculated outrageousness, that isn't a bad score.) In my sixties, I find I lose three friends to every friend I gain. Some are lost to death. In a few cases, I have made a deliberate attempt to cut back friendships that go back to my high school days — as I noted, I live in the city in which I grew up, so my urban landscape is dotted with fifty- or sixty-year acquaintanceships — having decided that some of these no longer have any real content for me.

Another class of old friend has arisen at this stage in my life: a man or woman I like well enough but have no strong desire to see. I am glad to hear from them, on the phone or through e-mail, but at the close of our exchange there is a slightly embarrassed moment that would normally be filled in by mention of getting together for lunch or coffee, but now, when I permit my good sense to outweigh my sentimentality, is not.

Despite my desire to trim down the number of my friendships, I find I continue to enter into new, much valued ones. I have by now a too firmly ingrained cordiality, and find I cannot, even if I try, put up a cold façade. (Only my heart, I can hear some readers of this chapter say, remains cold.) Not long before writing this, I ended my university teaching, and one of the secret pleasures of doing so is that it means I shall no longer fall in love, in the platonic sense, with any more students.

With adults, the criteria for being a friend of mine become less certain. Three or so years ago, I was told by a friend, a mathematician, that a friend of hers, also a mathematician, was an admirer of my writing and that he and his wife would like one day to meet me and my wife. We met in a noisy Italian restaurant on the North Side of Chicago, and I found my heart going out to this man and his wife five minutes after introductions.

On the surface, we had little in common except that we were of the same generation. He is a man without physical vanity, while mine is substantial; the caste of his mind is scientific and logical, while mine is literary and intuitive. We shared no professional interests. Although they have lived in America for more than twenty-five years, he and his wife were raised in Israel, and I have not had great luck in my relations with Israelis; their political seriousness is greater than mine, their taste for whimsy less, and they tend, in my experience, to disregard the many subtleties in friendships and details in daily pleasures that for me are of the greatest interest. And yet, in that crowded restaurant, I sensed that I wanted to see this man and his kind-hearted wife again.

And I have since done so, with a deepening sense of affection and closeness. Shared laughter has been a good part of the reason, but this needs to be qualified: we laugh — he explosively, I gigglingly — at the arbitrariness, orneriness, goofiness, sweetness, perversity, generosity, self-absorption, and magnanimity of human beings, qualities that, taken together, make plain the hopelessness of the prospect of ever solving the puzzle of what constitutes human nature. He has easy access to what I do (write stories and essays); I have none whatsoever to what he does (mathematics and the training of future mathematicians). He is generous about my work; I am quiet, not to say dumbfounded, about his. My status in the world is probably slightly higher than his, while his accomplishments, I strongly suspect, are greater than mine: among other things, as a young man he was an Israeli army officer and faced death in battle; I was a draftee who wrote movie reviews in Texas and typed up the results of physical examinations in Arkansas.

We are both Jewish, my Jewishness being more secular (and ignorant) than his. I am three years older than he; and though we are contemporaries, our not having had a common background tends to nullify this element in our friendship: we cannot talk baseball together, or high school adventures, or what the city we both live in was like when we were boys. Without ever having to say so, we know that what we have in common is a congruent point of view of the human comedy — and it is more than enough.

Can I count on his loyalty, or he on mine? Neither of us can know for sure, but my instincts tell me that I could count on him. He is, I believe, distinctly a man for my foxhole — and for my dinner table. He doesn't suffer fools gladly, if at all. Would my having opinions he thought unacceptable put him off me? I don't know that either, except I believe that, faced with such an opinion from me, he would want to know why I held it before dismissing me as idiotic; I would, in other words, get a fair hearing from him. Ours is a friendship, let me here add, that has thus far never been tested, and I hope that it never will be. And why, after all, need it be?

Which leads me to what ought to seem obvious, but until this moment hasn't seemed obvious at all to me: the criteria for friendship can be set down only in so rough a way that they are all but useless. One might begin by saying that one's friends must be honorable, fair, decent, good-humored, generous, and kind. But inevitably some of one's dearest friends won't quite pass the test. They will have some of these qualities, or one or two in sufficiently attractive form, to make up for not having the others, or perhaps have them only in short supply. Nor, if the truth be known, is oneself (and myself) likely to possess the criteria of virtue required by the perfect friend.

The English philosopher Michael Oakeshott underscores this when he writes that "to discard friends because they do not behave as we expected and refuse to be educated to our requirements is the conduct of a man who has altogether mistaken the character of friendship." He continues: "Friends are not concerned with what might be made of one another, but only with the enjoyment of one another: and the condition of this enjoyment is a ready acceptance of what is and the absence of any desire to change or improve." A friend, he adds, is "somebody who engages the imagination, who excites contemplation, who provokes interest, sympathy, delight and loyalty simply on account of the relation entered into." Oakeshott ends by writing that "the relationship of friend to friend is dramatic, not utilitarian; the tie is one of familiarity, not usefulness."

From which two points arise: First, friendship is almost never ideal, and imposing ideal standards on it is almost always a poor idea. Second, we enter into friendships largely through instinct — something about this man or woman that I like, though I can't at the moment say exactly what it is — and find our reasons for our attraction to them in an ad hoc or improvised and after-the-fact way. (In this, it is like love.) Few things are likelier to kill a friendship quicker than a careful and strictly adhered-to theory of what qualities are needed in a friend.

# 5

❖

# *Friends —*
# *Who Needs 'Em?*

"FOR WITHOUT FRIENDS," writes Aristotle, in the *Ethics,* "no one would choose to live." Aristotle goes on from here to run the categories of those who need friends: The prosperous and successful need them to exercise their beneficence, and also to guard and help preserve their wealth. In poverty and misfortune, Aristotle claims, friends are the only refuge. Friends help keep the young from error, and help the older by ministering to their needs and shoring up their weaknesses as life winds down; and friends lead those in the prime of life to contemplate noble deeds that will win approbation.

These are all rather utilitarian reasons for friendship. Aristotle was of course born well before the age of self-regarding psychology, and so was less likely to dive down to the darker waters of hidden motives behind friendship. Do we look to friends, for example, for self-affirmation — that is, to affirm our own best evaluation of ourselves — or, in the cant phrase of the day, to pump up our self-esteem? Is friendship, when stripped down to its essentials, just another playing field for that insatiably greedy and sleepless monster, the human ego? A comic line of our time runs, "It's always about you, isn't it?" Does friendship qualify here, too? Is it, finally, always about "me" or "you" — about, in other words, little more than making me or you feel good?

One would like to say, without hesitation, absolutely not to all these questions. But consider. In its broadest lineaments, the argument that friendship is chiefly about self-affirmation holds that none of us exists outside a social context. Our sense of our own value, in this reading, is almost wholly dependent on what others think of us. Obviously, most of us are pleased to count as friends people of whose high opinion of us we can be certain. (No one but a certified masochist could bear a friendship with someone who is always putting down or otherwise deflating him.) If we have noble or generous or impressive achievements in our past, it's pleasing to think that the people with whom we are friendly know about these things. Pleasing, too, even late in life, to be in a group where many people know that one was once a good athlete, physically beautiful, a great student, a solid parent, a fine provider, a splendid person all around. Among friends, one doesn't have to establish afresh one's bona fides about one's real quality.

Do we take our conception of ourselves from outside ourselves, the question is, or are we strong enough to know our true value without seeing it reflected in the eyes of friends? Some writers, artists, and composers have known they were good, superior even, without any signs of their quality being registered in criticism, the marketplace, or the estimation of people who love them: Henri Matisse, Stéphane Mallarmé, James Joyce, Arnold Schoenberg come to mind. Of their own quality they were without doubt; and, among a small number of such people — many of them avant-garde geniuses — they required no other valuation than self-knowledge, which informed their unwavering high opinion of themselves. (Exceptions to this exist in the arts, of course: Virginia Woolf, judging from her diaries, seemed to have been in a state of near-permanent insecurity about the quality of her art and of endless worry about what the people who mattered to her thought about it.) But are there many people outside the arts who have the same confidence?

My father seems to have been such a person. He was a good, gentle, generous, fair man, yet in all the time I knew him, a man without anything resembling friends. When I was a boy, if the phone rang in our apartment, my father would joke that if it was for him — the joke here is that it never was — to tell the party calling that he had left the country. My father had friends as a boy and as a young man, but once he married and found the work that he was able to devote himself to, friendships seemed to hold no real allure for him. Such social life as he had was with the husbands of my mother's friends, and he never went beyond a middling sociability with any of them. In place of friends, he had family; in place of a social life, he had his business. The people who came closest to being his friends were those he knew through work, but he rarely saw them in the evening or on weekends.

My father's fairly high valuation of himself was owing to his having made a small but genuine success at his business. Born a Canadian, he moved to Chicago when he was seventeen, without finishing high school. Such social life as he had centered on his extended family. He played no cards, felt golf a game for morons, understood that country and city clubs could never be his milieu. He had a marriage in which his wife was his best friend. He could be courtly without being unduly formal, and he had a good sense of humor, but he had no great gift for intimacy. He apparently had no need for masculine company. He wasn't especially antisocial. (He was, in the 1940s, briefly a Mason.) Had you met him, you would not, I think, disagree with a description of him as "cordial." Never was it a question of his having lost, or longed for, friends; he simply didn't require them, and so never bothered to acquire them. And, as his son, and someone who knew him for more than sixty years, I cannot say that he ever seemed to miss them.

My father had a firm sense of himself as a serious and productive and independent person. He was filled with opinions about human nature and the way the world worked; though he didn't force them on anyone, neither could he quite hold them back. (He had developed the art of the falsely modest introductory clause: "I could be wrong about this, of course . . ." "This is just off the top of my head, but I'm inclined to think . . .") As a self-made man, he felt he had some authority to speak about the world; and as far as I was concerned, he did have the authority, if not always anywhere near enough to support his heady theories about demography and war, the various hidden purports of Mother Nature, and the like.

His success at his business may have conferred on him all the self-regard he needed. Having friends in important places, having someone besides his wife to confide in, having people with whom he could be utterly relaxed and himself, none of these things seemed to matter to him. He wanted to be thought an agreeable person, but I don't think he cared all that much if someone found him otherwise. He was what he was — which is to say, he was always himself. Inner-directed, in David Riesman's once famous scheme of psychological types, is what my father was, and to a high degree.

While my mother was my father's best friend, I'm far from certain that he was *her* best friend, though her love for him was constant and without qualification. Owing to his temperament and his total absorption in his work, he could not hope to come close to supplying her with her social requirements. My mother was a very sociable woman. She always had circles of friends, belonged to card-playing groups, and went to lots of luncheons and charity events of the kind that women of her generation called "affairs." Nor had she the least snobbery. Her only qualification for a friend, so far as I can determine, was that she have a good heart, which my mother herself had. Thus she became friends with the woman, an immigrant who survived Hitler's death camps, who began as her seamstress, and sometimes she would spend mornings with this woman, listening to her stories about life in Poland, and Saturday mornings my mother drove her around on shopping errands.

As a married man, I resemble my father in having, as my best friend, my wife. But I also have a knack — a flaw perhaps is better — for a too easy intimacy, described earlier, that leads some people to believe that I want to be closer to them than I actually do. People mistake friendliness in me for friendship, two quite distinct things. Because of this, I suspect that the number of people in the world who might call me a good friend is larger than the number of people I would claim as good friends.

When I ask myself what my friends do for me, I find myself retreating into vapidities. With friends I feel the comfort of a common outlook — amused, ironic, not altogether unhappy to be slightly out of it as we grow older together. More than anything else I find comfort in my close friends: an easiness that allows me to be myself. Not, I hasten to add, that I have several alternative selves available to me to be. I pride myself on having arrived at an age when pretense seems silly, if not comical. (My general style, once perhaps carefully cultivated, but now quite real, is that of being a man reasonably at ease in the world.) Yet with these few friends, I can, so to say, be even more myself: risk wild allusiveness, drop diplomacy, heighten candor. Knowing how their sense of humor works, I can play on my own with a spontaneity and freedom that I can't generally call into play with lesser friends. These close friends and I do not agree on everything — only on important, only on the main, things.

I hope I don't need reinforcement from friends for such ideas as I have, such opinions as I hold, such core beliefs as I expect to die with. Agreement in these and other matters can of course cushion friendship, removing the potholes and bumpy places all friendships of any duration encounter. I have met many people whose opinions were vastly different from my own, and discovered that this deprived them neither of charm nor, when I permitted myself to gaze beyond their mere opinions, of my affection.

On the other side, I've met people many of whose opinions are nearly congruent with my own whom I find entirely objectionable and wouldn't want to be with for the time it takes to drink a cup of coffee. When I lived in Little Rock, Arkansas, in the early and middle sixties, all friendships were formed on the basis of one's views on racial integration. I had acquaintances who were not integrationists, but my social circle was made up exclusively of people who were for racial integration (not so obvious or easy a thing to be openly for in Arkansas in those years, especially if one happened to have been born in the South). Yet in those days I often thought how, but for this single matter of enlightened opinions about race, I would not choose to spend much time with many of these people, and, after I moved out of the South, our interest in one another lapsed and fell away. These were, in effect, single-issue friendships, which are not usually built to last.

Over the years I have had friends connected with specific activities: tennis friends, racquetball friends, poker friends. But when the games were over, so too, until the next session of games, were the friendships. As I have grown older, many of my friendships have come to have distinct limits. I have a friend, from our days in the army together, with whom I went to one Chicago Cubs game a year, until he moved to Virginia. I have another friend whom I meet with for lunch precisely twice a year: once in spring, once in the fall. If I see a friend, even a good friend, on Wednesday, I'm likely to arrange things so that I don't see him or her again on Friday. If this all sounds rather cold and calculating, this is only because it is — or at least it's calculating.

When I am with certain friends, I am, variously, content, amused, happy, sometimes all these things at once. But I do not mentally crave the pleasures of friendship as once I did. Too often I feel, more than straightforward affection, a corroding sense of obligation; and as the sociologist Ray Pahl puts it, "if we feel obliged to be a friend, then it is no true friendship." Nietzsche said that to live alone, a man must be a god or a beast. I know I am not the first, and hope I'm not turning into the second. Is it that much of my former need for friends is now supplied by my wife, a person many of whose interests and much of whose point of view are so close to my own? Is it that, having grown older, I have come to enjoy solitude more?

In an introduction to Jocelyn Brooke's Orchid Trilogy, Anthony Powell writes of his friendship with Brooke: "I was never a close friend of Jocelyn Brooke's, but we corresponded quite often, and he was one of the people to whom one wrote letters with great ease. He speaks more than once of his own liking for that sort of relationship, a kind that did not make him feel hemmed in. There are several incidents in his books when the narrator refuses an invitation from someone with whom he is getting on pretty well so that it was no great surprise when, a few months after Brooke had stayed with us for a weekend, he politely excused himself from another visit on grounds of work. The reason may have been valid enough, writing time is always hard to conserve, but one suspected his sense of feeling 'different,' unwillingness to cope with face-to-face cordialities of a kind that might at the same time be agreeable in letters." I am not so odd as Jocelyn Brooke, but I have come to a time in life when I can understand his oblique motives.

I sometimes feel my life too crowded with friends, of various kinds. Some contemporaries among my friends have reached the stage of ceasing to listen, but only wait to speak, which they often do about things I have heard them say more than twice before. With them meetings are no longer as pleasant as I remember them having been: the laughter is less, the flow of talk not as spirited, the glow of good feeling afterward occasionally nonexistent.

Friendship, in other words, can come to seem a burden. I want friends, yes, but I want them at my convenience: the right ones at the right time. This is a condition of course that can be met only by what were once known as call girls, and friends, quite rightly, won't — and shouldn't — stand for it. Still . . .

Why are people drawn to me? Embarrassing question though it is to confront, I would say it is due in part to the general aura, the high-octane fumes, of friendliness I often give off, to the promise my personality seems to hold out for charm and chumminess: I am teller of jokes, a doubtless too frequent reteller of well-polished anecdotes, someone who attempts to use language in an amusing way. But I also think that I come off — I say "come off," which is, please note, different from "am" — as someone who is comfortable in his own skin, not vulnerable or needy, a man who is sailing through life well in control, owing to his strong sense of autonomy. Whether this is actually so is perhaps not a question for me to answer.

What if, reading the above paragraphs, my friends — many of whom are happily without knowledge of one another's existence — were to hold a meeting in which they established an easily arrived at consensus to abandon me? What would my life be like without friends?

Undoubtedly poorer — much poorer. My relationship with my wife, however dear to me, cannot supply all my social needs. Although she is a highly cultured woman, some of my intellectual pursuits are outside her realm of interest. She knows only a minimum about my professional dealings with magazine and book editors, literary agents and publishers. I am more vulgar than she, with a number of small but real passions — for sports, unhealthy food, off-color jokes (not too off-color; roughly turquoise, I'd say) — that I am just as glad she doesn't share. Although she is the only person in the world with whom I can speak freely — not always easily, but freely — about things of the heart, she cannot be all things for me, and I know I cannot be all things for her.

I retain friends for various of these (I wish there were a better word than the one I am about to use) needs. With some friends of my own age I can talk about how goofy the world has become — and how different from the world in which we grew up. With others I can talk in a detailed way about mildly abstract things: politics, the current state of the university, the quality of literary and intellectual life. With still others I can talk about brutish things: sports, the comedy of sex, and use such charming words as mother-grabber and nice boobs.

This begins to sound sour — the plaint of a man claiming he is surfeited by friendship, a thing too many people are forced to do without and long to have. Is this condition of surfeit exclusive to me — is it solipsism and little more — or does it have to do with the modern nature of friendship in lives that have come to seem altogether too crowded?

As a scribbling man, a writer, I have come not only to accept but to appreciate, even enjoy, being alone. This appreciation may have a good deal to do with why I chose a writing life to begin with. Replying to the young Desmond MacCarthy, who asked him why he chose to become a writer, Henry James wrote: "The port from which I set out was, I think, that of the *essential loneliness of my life* — and it seems to me the port, in sooth, to which again finally my course directs itself. This loneliness (since I mention it) — what is it still but the deepest thing about one? Deeper about me, at any rate, than anything else, deeper than my 'genius,' deeper than my 'discipline,' deeper than any pride, deeper above all than the deep counter-minings of art." Not to compare myself with the masterly Henry James, but I have felt such loneliness, too. One doesn't need to be a writer to feel it.

Georg Simmel, the always penetrating German sociologist, believed that modern society tended to undermine soulful friendships of the kind that Aristotle espoused, and that with the twentieth century new forms of friendship had emerged, which he termed "differentiated friendships." In *The Secret Society,* Simmel wrote:

> These differentiated friendships which connect us with one individual in terms of affection, with another in terms of intellectual aspects, with a third in terms of religious impulses, and with a fourth in terms of common experiences — all these friendships present a very peculiar synthesis in regard to the question of discretion, of reciprocal revelation and concealment. They require that the friends do not look into those mutual spheres of interest and feeling which, after all, are not included in the relation and which, if touched upon, would make them feel painfully the limits of their mutual understanding.

Simmel is saying that friendship has become specialized and fragmented. Friends have come to resemble nothing so much as wardrobe: one puts on different ones for different occasions. The all-purpose, deep-relationship friend, of the kind Aristotle vaunted and that Montaigne found in Étienne de La Boétie, is, Simmel asserts, no longer available to modern men and women; we have "too much to hide to sustain a friendship in the ancient sense" — a friendship that, in Simmel's words, connected "a whole person with another in [his or her] entirety; . . . the modern way of feeling tends more heavily toward differentiated feelings."

Is the problem, then, linked to this new kind of — these differentiated — friends? Has modern life changed the very nature of friendship, so that many of us feel alternately lonely or else hemmed in by the demands of friends? Or has true friendship always been a tender shoot, a fragile and difficult thing to sustain? Perhaps La Rochefoucauld, that most thoroughgoing of cynics, was correct when he wrote: "However rare true love may be, it is less so than true friendship."

# 6

❖

# *An Extremely Sketchy History of Friendship*

So FAR AS I KNOW, nothing exists in the way of organized histories of friendship in any of the major cultures or countries of the West or East. No doubt this is owing to the multiplicity and complexity of friendly relations, or what the philosopher Galen Strawson has called "the large untidy essence" of friendship. Historically, friendship is a subject much taken for granted and one often lost in the politically more potent and more significant matter of relationships formed for pacts, alliances, and conspiracies. Perhaps it is best that there is no thorough history of friendship; the comprehensiveness required would make for a backachingly dull book. Still, the subject does have a historical dimension, for friendship, in its nature and its forms, has changed in various ways over the centuries.

The Bible is not rife with stories of friendship, and only two stand out: that between Jonathan and David and that between Ruth and Naomi. Jonathan was forced to dance the tightrope between loyalty to a friend (David) and devotion to a father (Saul), and, operating under great pressure, was able to do so with reasonable success. The friendship between Ruth and Naomi gave us the beautiful verse that runs: "Whither thou goest, I will go; and where thou lodgest, I will lodge; thy people shall be my people, and thy God my God; where thou diest, will I die, and there will I be buried; the Lord do so to me and more also, if aught but death part thee and me." This verse, said by a friend to a friend, is nowadays mostly used in marriage ceremonies and is thought to represent the commitment that successfully flows from romantic love. One could draw from this the point that what was once thought to be fealty of a kind owed to friendship is now being asked for marriage. The Old Testament is otherwise thin on friendship. For the most part, it is about family, which means dynasties, rivalries (sibling and other), complicated marriages, endless fallings-out.

The New Testament is even thinner. "Christian love teaches love of all men, unconditionally all," wrote Søren Kierkegaard. "Let the poet search the New Testament for a word about friendship which could please him, and he will search vainly unto despair." The problem is that friendship is particular and exclusionary; Christianity, in its intention at least, is universal and all-embracing. As Gillian and Stephen R. L. Clark report in their contribution to a book of essays by various hands called *The Dialects of Friendship,* one is unlikely "to find an entry under 'Friendship' in dictionaries of Christian thought or Christian ethics," to which they add that "Christian thinking about friendship is part of a wider preoccupation with proper human — and creaturely — relationships."

"Greater love hath no man than this," it is written in the book of John (15:13), "that he lay down his life for his friends." But much more life is laid down for friends in classical than in biblical times. In Greek mythology, there are the famous friendships between Theseus and Perithous, Damon and Pythias, Orestes and Pylades. The great friendship in Homeric Greece is that between Achilles and his brother-in-law and beloved friend Patroclus. But this famous friendship seems a one-way concern, with Patroclus, though the elder of the two, used by Achilles as something of a gofer. He is told, for example, to return the maiden Briseis to King Agamemnon. After Patroclus is slain by Hector, his death furnishes the reason for Achilles' devastating rage. Patroclus requested of Achilles that "a single urn, the gold two-handled urn your noble mother gave you, hold our bones — together." Achilles accedes to the request, and goes well beyond it in setting up astonishing funeral rites for his friend Patroclus after his own revenging slaughter of Hector. But his vengeance is for "my dear comrade's death . . . the man I loved beyond all other comrades, loved as my own life—I've lost him." Friendship, then, quite as much as the beautiful face of Helen, may be said to have brought down Troy.

Both *The Iliad* and *The Odyssey* were composed in the eighth century B.C., and after that friendships in Greek culture, at least from the predominating Athenian point of view, appear less emphasized than great solitary figures—Solon, Pericles, Alcibiades—who seem to spring into their greatness without the contrivance of friends and allies, as political figures do later in Rome, but through the force of their character and oratorical and political gifts. Socrates, who claimed many friends, was too far superior a man to have anything like intimate friends among them. Who, after all, could be his equal in virtue? In Athens, family remained of first significance. Family could sometimes entail a complex friend-like relation with families from other city-states, known as *xenos,* in which loyalty of a highly qualified kind was felt to be owed between families.

In Sparta, where community was emphasized above family, so much so that children were communally raised and meals were eaten in a common mess, friendship perhaps loomed larger than family. We have the notable—and noble—story of the three hundred Spartan soldiers, comrades in the deepest sense, who held off thousands of Persians at Thermopylae. Male Spartan youths went through the rigorous training known as the *agōgē,* in which men between the ages of twenty and thirty trained young boys in the arts of war. Friendships must have been formed, but so stern was the training, in which the group took precedence over all else, that the formation of friendship was unlikely to have been the first order of business. Whether the relationships between older and younger men in Spartan society were pederastic is, among scholars, a matter still in the flux of controversy.

As in the modern era, friendship among the Greeks implied loyalty, a certain rough reciprocity, good faith, altruism, and unselfish affection, all apart from the realms of business and politics. "Never in antiquity," David Konstan writes in *Friendship in the Classical World,* "so far as I am aware, is the revelation of personal intimacies described as necessary to the formation of friendship." Konstan adds that "in classical Greece erotic love [between men] and friendship were understood normally to be incomplete relationships." Sophocles thought that between loyalty to one's city-state and one's friends there could be no contest: one's city-state took clear and obvious precedence.

Much is made of the friendship of Alexander the Great and Hephaestion, "dearest of all his friends." Many think that Alexander, who may be said to have suffered something like an Achilles complex, used the death of his friend to express an Achilles-like grief. But insofar as friendship for the Greeks implied equality, no one, finally, could truly have been Alexander's friend, for he was, in all senses of the word, peerless.

Epicurus (341–270 B.C.), the founder of the school of Epicureans, featured friendship in his plan for the good life. Much maligned by the Stoics and other rivaling schools for their reputed hedonism, the Epicureans in fact believed in reducing life to its simplest elements, Epicurus himself saying he was content with water and barley bread. Epicurus bought a house in Athens with an ample garden in which he installed his followers, who were known for the warmth of their friendship. Epicurus himself was said to have been in every way a good and solicitous friend. "Only beasts," he claimed, "dine alone."

The Epicureans were united by a code of moral conduct that held, essentially, that pleasure in life came not from satisfying desires but from eliminating anxieties. The most efficient way of achieving this, Epicurus stated, was not to fear God or death (which merely brought oblivion, a *tabula rasa* state like that before our birth), and to limit our desires to the necessary and remember that even terrible pain figures to be short-lived. He also believed that happiness entailed withdrawal from public life, at that time a most un-Greek notion. In this scheme, Epicurus held friendship to be among life's necessities, and his truly was a community of friends. "Friendship," he wrote, "dances around the world announcing that we must wake up to blessedness." The only shortcoming was that Epicurus was himself admired by his followers to the point of adoration, and among his circle no criticism of his doctrines was permitted.

With the Romans, friendship takes a political, or utilitarian, turn. The Latin word for friendship, *amicitia*, is said to have had its origin in party politics. In Rome marriage had a strong political element, with husband and wife forming an alliance of sorts in a world where political intrigue was pervasive. Friendship was inextricably linked to utility, which, it will be recalled, Aristotle did not rank highly.

Marcus Tullius Cicero (106–43 B.C.) was a man of many friendships and himself the author of one of the central texts on friendship, called *Laelius de Amicitia*. Not highborn but a so-called "new man," Cicero was both brilliant and vain, noble of spirit and cowardly. Volatile in his passions, he was ambitious and acquisitive, made bad marriages, overrated his children, was ruinously prodigal, with a special weakness for real estate (he was house-proud) and art works, and nothing if not contentious — he begins to sound, as this description suggests, like the first modern man.

The specialty of the Romans in philosophy was applied morality. The place of the passions, the ranking of life's duties, the pressures placed on virtue in political life, the likely future after death — these were Cicero the philosopher's principal subjects. To give but a brief sample of the impressive specificity of Cicero's thinking, here he is on the subject of friendship put to the test of politics: "It is not in human nature to be indifferent to political power; and if the price men have to pay for it is the sacrifice of friendship, they think their treason will be thrown into the shade by the magnitude of the reward. This is why friendship is very difficult to find among those who engage in politics and the contest for office. Where can you find the man to prefer his friend's advancement to his own? And to say nothing of that, think how grievous and almost intolerable it is to most men to share political disaster." Cicero, like Montaigne much later, could gear up the ideal of friendship quite high, defining it as "nothing other than agreement over all things divine and human along with good will and affection."

Cicero's dearest friend was Titus Pomponius Atticus, a wealthy businessman with a taste for literary pursuits and book collecting and with a knack for avoiding political intrigue — no easy task in Rome during the time of the transition between the fall of the Roman republic and the beginning of the empire. Because Cicero's letters to Atticus have survived, we know much about Cicero's relations with friends and about the way he made use of them. Cicero went to Atticus for financial advice and aid, on personal matters (a discussion of prospective second wives for Cicero is one of their subjects), and for endless discussions of the perilous political situations in which his equivocal ambitions landed him.

Cicero also went to Atticus to rehearse his troubles. Living in exile, Cicero reports to his friend about his loss of weight and propensity for weeping, and adds: "Has any man ever fallen from so fine a position, with so good a cause, so strong in resources of talent, prudence and influence, and in the support of all honest men? Can I forget what I was or fail to feel what I am and what I have lost — rank, fame, children, fortune, brother?"

This note of confession will of course play a larger and larger role in friendship in our own day — a day that has seen what I think it accurate to call the triumph of the therapeutic, in which a friend, as like as not several friends, serve one another as surrogate psychotherapists, to whom to recount disappointments, secrets, troubles little and large, so that the word "intimacy," so long associated with friendship, has also become nearly synonymous with "confessional."

One hundred and fifty years later, in the letters of Gaius Plinius Caecilius Secundus (A.D. 61–c. 112), better known as Pliny the Younger, one sees friendship under the Roman Empire in full bloom, and much of it seems to turn on what we today call networking. A conscientious friend, Pliny seems always busy making connections for other friends: advising this friend to give the son of that friend a job, arranging a teacher for the nephew of another friend, from time to time doing a bit of matchmaking between the children of friends. Pliny the Younger was full of praise for his friends. He writes to one Minicius Fundanas in support of another friend, Asinius Rufus, that Rufus is also the close friend of Cornelius Tacitus (the great historian), "and you know the sort of man Tacitus is. So, if you think highly of us both, you should think highly of Rufus, since there is no bond in friendship stronger than similarity of character."

Pliny was an operator, but insofar as one can determine, most of the time an operator with no ulterior motive. He was an impressive broker of favors who chiefly wished to do well by his friends and his friends' children, and who also saw friendship in the context of Roman concepts of justice and honor.

Christianity, with its command to love all persons, even one's enemies — "This is my command," said Jesus, "that you love one another as I have loved you" — may be, at least obliquely, anti-friendship; for friendship, as remarked earlier, is by its nature exclusive and excluding, and Christianity democratic and all-inclusive. The Good Samaritan did not reserve his good works for his friends but expended them without discrimination on anyone in need. If one must love one's enemies, that doesn't leave much left over for one's friends, though some dispute a too strict reading of this credo. ("He who loves his enemies betrays his friends; / This surely is not what Jesus intends," wrote William Blake.) None of this is to say that one cannot be a good Christian and value particular friendships; only that friendship per se is not emphasized in doctrinal Christianity.

Saint Augustine quotes Cicero's treatise on friendship in *The City of God,* where Cicero seems to worry about the stabs of betrayal that friendship might bring rather than to praise the glories of friendship. In this work Augustine advises that we should be pleased when good friends die before they "have fallen from faith or from moral conflict — that is, that they have died in their very soul." In *The Confessions,* he speaks of losing a best friend from the days when he was still a young man and had not yet found his religious vocation. He lost this friend — whose name he does not give — only a little after they were together for a year.

As with Montaigne in his friendship with La Boétie, Augustine is much longer on his grief than on setting out the precise nature of the pleasures of the friendship; he even sounds like Montaigne when he writes: "I was surprised that other mortals were alive, since that when he whom I had loved was dead I was still alive, for he was my 'other self.' Someone has well said of his friend, 'He was half my soul.'" (Augustine is here quoting Horace on Virgil in the *Odes*.) John Milton made famous his friendship with Edward King (1612–1637)—who died, at twenty-five, in the North Channel off Ireland—in his poem "Lycidas." It begins to seem that the most efficient way to qualify as one of history's elite circle of best friends is to be chums briefly with a great writer when you are both young and then have the good sense to peg out well before you turn forty.

But throughout history one realizes how rare is the perfect friend. Cicero says, truly, that "most people unreasonably . . . want such a friend as they are unable to be themselves, and expect from their friends what they do not themselves give." He also offers this sensible but useless piece of advice: take "such care in the selection of friends as never to enter upon a friendship with a man whom we could under any circumstances come to hate." He speaks of allowing friendships to die naturally, through inanition. But a great many friendships, as we know, end otherwise, leaving regret, rancor, resentment, sadness all around. Whom better to hate, after all, than someone one has formerly loved. (Colette holds the reverse position, finding that to love someone whom one formerly despised is the most emotionally delicious of all.)

Some things have remained constant through the history of friendship, among them the notion that one will be judged by the company, or friendships, one keeps. In the early sixteenth century Baldassare Castiglione, the author of *The Book of the Courtier*, writes of the care that is required in choosing friends: "There is another thing which seems to me to create or take away from reputation, and this is our choice of the friends with whom we are to live in intimate relations; for reason doubtless requires that persons who are joined in close friendship and in indissoluble companionship must be alike in their minds, their judgments, and talents. Thus, he who associates with the ignorant or the wicked is held to be ignorant or wicked; and, on the contrary, he who associates with the good, the wise, and the discreet is taken to be such himself. For it seems that everything naturally and readily joins with its like." And so, then as now, the moral is clear: you are judged by the company you keep.

The German sociologist Ferdinand Tönnies and other theoreticians of capitalism viewed the new organization of society required by industrialization and urbanization as taking its toll on friendship, with market relations — including longer working hours, crowded conditions, social-class segregation — often taking precedence over normally personal ones. Others, among them Alexis de Tocqueville, stressing the importance of voluntary associations (church membership, trade unions, cooperative groups) in modern life, saw them as places where friendships of a new and different order were made.

More recently, though, there is a feeling — certainly it is my feeling — that something further has changed. One sees this argument in Digby Anderson's *Losing Friends.* "If we ask ourselves," Anderson writes, "whether there are a significant number of people today without true friends, or whether our modern society is one in which friendship plays a diminishing role, I think the answers are yes."

Digby Anderson writes as a strong yet saddened advocate of friendship, which he believes is in a bad way. Friendship is, he rightly holds, a relationship without a legal status, so that, for example, if a man dies intestate, his assets would go not to the dear friend or friends who may have taken good care of him for years right up to the end, but instead quite possibly to a distant relative whom the deceased may never have met.

Anderson also feels that much modern friendship has been knocked askew by therapeutic notions that posit human beings as almost continually changing: plant-like, we seem, in the popular botanical metaphor, always growing. Thus it is that people feel they need different friends at different stages in their lives. (Sometimes, for much the same reasons, different husbands and wives, too.) In a therapeutic age, perpetually changing personality (with its needs for endless growth, change, self-esteem) trumps solidly built friendships based on unchanging character every time.

Mobility, which entails people moving from city to city owing to their jobs, or seeking the sun in their retirement, or fresh new starts in life, also cuts into friendship. Divorce, itself a form of social mobility and now all too common, can also destroy friendships, especially those sweet miracles of four- (or more) way reciprocity involving two (or more) couples, all getting on beautifully with one another until divorce causes it all to collapse.

Digby Anderson also sees fewer social institutions dedicated to same-sex friendship (especially among men) and a diminishing of attraction in those that not so long ago were strong: men's clubs, pub life, fraternities and sororities of the kind of the Masons, the Knights of Columbus, church sodalities, and the rest. In a more and more privatized world, friendship is for spare time; it has become less central to life and increasingly recreational, like croquet or poker.

In some ways, one of the greatest enemies of friendship is the family as we have come to conceive it over the past forty or so years. Often one feels closer to friends than one does to brothers and sisters. Yet, ironically, one of the few ways we have to describe the intensity of friendships is to say of a friend that "he is like a brother to me," or "she is like a member of the family."

In a highly child-centered society, where above all "attention must be paid" to children, friendship cannot hope to compete. Where friendship requires sacrifice, which usually entails spending time in aiding friends, it is everywhere understood that this must not cut too deeply into time ("quality time," in the clichéd phrase) spent with family. Even when one no longer has children in the home, the claims of friendship remain at best secondary to those of family, including, increasingly, to the duties of caring for aging parents or young grandchildren. Ought one, say, to go off for a week or more with a few friends of one's own sex when one's husband or wife has first claim on one's attention? The answer is obvious.

Today anyone who suggested that a friend ought to come before a wife would be thought more than a little nuts and soon likely to be in need of the services of a divorce lawyer. In any competition between friendship and marriage, friendship loses every time. Charles Lamb touches on this point in his essay "A Bachelor's Complaint," suggesting that, in his experience, the good friend of the groom is lucky if he lasts in his old condition of closeness for more than twelve months after the marriage.

It is a great advantage in life to love one's husband or wife, and the greatest marriages are those in which husband and wife, along with being lovers, in the fullness of time become best friends. But these marriages tend, if not to dampen, then at least to detract from friendships. With a wife or husband who is truly one's Étienne de La Boétie or Titus Pomponius Atticus, with physical love and the mutual interest in one's children added, one requires less in and from other friends. Sometimes, in fact, when one has such a dominant best friend — a live-in, as it were, best friend — the expectations and obligations of other friendships can come to seem a touch, and sometimes more than a touch, burdensome.

When one was a boy or girl friendship seemed unalloyed pleasure. Youth may be the prelapsarian stage of friendship. As one grows older, one begins to feel the pressures of expectation and obligation that are part of serious friendship. Soon the notion of reciprocity — which Adam Smith thought, however loosely applied, was unreckonable in friendship — enters into friendly relations. Friendship also comes to include accepting oddities, weaknesses, social and intellectual limitations, and other flaws in friends, and this can be complicated by the fact that some of these — depression, self-absorption, confining illnesses, stupendous boringness — were not there when the friendship began decades before. Nor were they bargained for; a friend is not, like a wife or husband, a permanent partner, in sickness and in health. Friendship, as those of us of a certain age learn, can grow much more complicated as one grows older.

"Unfortunate is the lot of that man who can look round the wide world and exclaim the truth, *I have no friend!*" wrote Charles Lamb in "Many Friends." "Do you know any such lonely sufferer? For mercy sake send him to me. I can afford him plenty." Lamb goes on to say that, owing to his temperament, he has way too many friends, is "positively pestered by friends." Lamb describes himself when writing this as "not old — a sort of middle-aged-gentleman-and-a-half," and his condition reminds me a little of my own. (I like to think Charles Lamb and I might have got on well, agreeing at the outset, of course, not to see each other with too great frequency.) Lamb's complaint is that, while society is truly "the balm of life," satiety in this line is easily reached. And I would say that in our time, when the calls on each of us are greater and greater, this seems even more true than in Lamb's day.

Nor do I wish to scamp the glories, indeed oftentimes astonishments, of friendship, which are genuine. Generosity is a strong element of friendship, and there is something saintly about the sweet desire of one friend wanting to make life more pleasant for another. Selflessness is high among the elements of true friendship, and selflessness implies the readiness to make sacrifices — not merely through the expression of love for one's friends, which is easy, but through what one is willing to do for them.

In so many of my current friendships I feel a sense of limitation. This, too, may be a sign of growing older, but also of the pressures of modern life, with its manifold claims on one's time. How far, I ask myself, would I go for the friends most dear to me? I have five or six friends who, if they came to me for a loan of, say, $50,000 for a medical emergency, I should find the money for them. I know perhaps a dozen people whom, if they wish to reveal to me that they find their regrets in life of much greater weight than their achievements, I should be willing to listen to, and offer whatever persuasive lies I could invent in the hope of providing them solace.

Has the nature of friendship, as I suspect, seriously, even fundamentally, changed? Have our lives, despite all the conveniences made possible by technology, become so crowded that in our day friendships can seem just as much an inconvenience as one of life's great pleasures? Is friendship, in an age when the therapeutic has triumphed, as uncomplicatedly satisfying as it once was?

Has the shifted interest in family and the extreme interest in child-rearing pushed friendship to a lower priority, something aside and apart, something secondary at best, reserved for leisure time? Can we any longer really lose ourselves in our friends, so that they become, in the classical formulation, "other selves" for whom we are prepared to sacrifice all and everything and upon whom we can count to do the same for us? Friendship, close friendship of the kind described by the classical writers, is an ideal as splendid as any set up by human beings, one charged by affection, generosity, and selflessness, but is this ideal still as available to us today as it once seemed to be?

# 7

❖

# *Reciprocity,*
# *or Is It Obligation?*

"T HE ACTIONS REQUIRED by friendship, humanity, hospitality generally are vague and indeterminate," wrote Adam Smith in *The Theory of Moral Sentiments.* Especially vague, I wish Adam Smith had added, are those connected with friendship. Many of these actions come under the heading of obligations. Whatever else it has to do with, friendship entails obligation—sometimes ample and demanding, sometimes minuscule and subtle, but always, I believe, present. In some friendships all the obligations seem to fall on one friend, which makes these friendships, on the face of it, flawed—one-sided friendships and therefore, in the nature of the case, unsatisfactory because unfair.

Often behind the obligations of friendship are the feelings associated with gratitude. One incurs the real debt of gratitude for acts of kindness, consideration, and generosity done to one, and unless one is inhuman, one feels grateful. "Gratitude," wrote Georg Simmel, "is the moral memory of mankind." Quite so. I used to joke that every family has its theme, and that of my parents was ingratitude: generous and good people, they nevertheless frequently felt that people on whom they had lavished their generosity and goodness were insufficiently grateful, to the point of sometimes cutting off old friendships, sometimes allowing them to sour and die. In many ways such behavior was out of character for them, but they seemed to be able to remember, vividly, every thank-you card they failed to receive.

I find I have to guard against fresh outbreaks of this family trait in myself. I send someone a book or article I have written and receive no response — it is duly noted. I help a former student make a connection that leads to his acquiring a job, and he thanks me in what I consider a perfunctory way — it is duly noted. I put myself out in some way for someone, I pick up a number of restaurant checks for someone else, I write something for a financially struggling magazine when I could get four or five times the fee it pays elsewhere, without any of these acts garnering what I consider proper thanks — noted, duly noted, all of it. None of this minor grievance-collecting brings me happiness, you understand; even permitting such thoughts makes me feel smaller of spirit; I wish to root such behavior out of myself. I can't claim, though, that I always succeed in doing so.

What obligations are owed me? What do I owe the many people who do out-of-the-ordinary things for me? Part of the difficulty is that these obligations are nowhere set out. Friendships have nothing resembling prenuptial contracts. Instead one deals, in a complex way, with equivalences. Am I doing my share, holding up my end of things, to keep this friendship intact?

Considering the obligations owed to genuine friends, at a minimum I should say that loyalty, or at least the absence of betrayal, is among them. Some press down on this quality harder than others. In some cultures, nothing less than fierce fidelity is demanded of friends; this is said to be so among Sicilians. In others, more latitude is permitted. Even here, though, things get a bit fuzzy. Is it permissible to speak of the oddities or weaknesses or flaws in one's friend while talking with another friend? Or does this constitute betrayal? If so, I have at one time or another probably betrayed most of my friends and, my guess is, many of my friends have betrayed me, and most people have similarly betrayed theirs.

Trust is often thought to be high among the obligations of modern friendship, but how far should it extend? Does trust in most friendships mean any more than goodwill? One hopes, for example, that in a situation where strangers might think poorly of you, friends will give you the benefit of every doubt. But we are flying without controls in trusting friends: no rules are laid down about limits. Ought friends with money in plentiful supply to lend us money when we need it? Such loans between friends, everyone has heard it said, are among the quickest ways to break up a friendship. Trust, too, is tricky terrain.

What about trusting friends with something greater than money: one's own vulnerabilities, doubts, disappointments, fears, terrors? Generally, we befriend people who operate at about the same level of discretion (or lack of discretion) as ourselves. Do you, for instance, really want to hear your friend tell you that her and her husband's sex life is a nightmare, details included? Would you want to hear a friend confess that he has been embezzling from his family business for years and feels rotten about it? Or that he has a strong dislike of his children? Or that she, entering into her seventh decade, feels her entire life a waste? Are these things friends can and should tell one another? Are they instead better told to a therapist? Or perhaps best kept to oneself, nicely suppressed in the name of dignified reticence?

The poet and philosopher Paul Valéry, one of the most introspective men who ever lived, wrote that "in general the things that people hide from each other are of an emotional or physiological nature, defects, manias, lusts, passions, and superstitions." He claimed that he himself had "only ever been able to confide in a single person who opened all the doors within me." That person, there is reason to believe, was not his wife but a late-life lover. Why do I feel I'd almost rather I didn't know that about this elegant and otherwise marvelously self-possessed man?

"A man, sir," said Dr. Johnson, "should keep his friendships in constant repair." By this I take Samuel Johnson to be saying that a man (or woman) should be aware of, and act upon, the obligations that friendship brings. One of the first of them, surely, is a certain regularity of meeting, at least when friends live in proximate distance of one another. The sociologists nowadays speak of "fossil friends" to refer to friends from one's geological past, from college, or high school days, or earlier, whom one can go without seeing for years and then pick up with roughly where you both left off. But a great many, probably most, friends are nongeological but on the surface of one's current life, and to let too much time lapse between visits with them is to suggest that one's interest in them is not genuine. The first obligation of friendship is attendance: one must plan and show up for meetings.

My own attendance with friends in recent years has fallen off. I have some friends I like a great deal whom I might not see for a yearlong stretch. I have others I might meet with every three months or so, still others I might meet every month. I have a dear friend with whom I generally speak over the phone at least once, often twice, a week, but four or five weeks might pass without our seeing each other in the flesh; and I haven't met him and his wife, in a foursome with my wife and me, for decades. I have some friends — I believe they qualify as friends — whom it pleases me to think about (all my memories of them are pleasant ones) but whom I nonetheless have almost no wish to be with. Among some of my friends, such is the fondness between us, even long distances between the cities in which we live do not seem to matter to the flow of our good feeling for each other, yet them I do long to see, and always leave them regretting that I may not do so for months or years.

Some attendance upon friends surely is compulsory. One ought to make a point of arranging to meet with a friend who has been seriously ill, or lost a close family member, or is undergoing true depression. Of course one ought. Friends in trouble need the solace of other friends; no surprise here. The notion of friends who were helpful in a difficult or sad time, or in a crisis, the notion that nowadays we account for by saying he or she was "there" for me, covers the point.

Or almost does. Not everyone wants even dear friends around or to fall back on at such times. I base this on the fact that, in difficult times in my own life, I seem not to have required such services of friends. Perhaps following in the path of my father, I discovered then, and still believe, that I prefer to

suffer my disappointments, setbacks, and failures alone, sometimes not mentioning the more minor among them to my wife,
to whom I can say almost anything, though there are things that
I cannot say to her and (I am sure) things she cannot—or
prefers not to—say to me. With rare exceptions, I think carrying on without (to invoke a new-fashioned word) "sharing" my
troubles is (to invoke a very old-fashioned word) "manly," possibly even dignified and graceful. In the spirit of the age, few
people, I realize, are likely to agree. Based on this passage, some
might conclude that I don't, and probably never have had, truly
close friends.

"Intimacy" has become one of the keystone words in defining a friend. The *Concise Oxford English Dictionary* definition,
given earlier, would seem to go along with this: a friend is "one
joined to another in intimacy and mutual benevolence independently of sexual or family love." But how to define "intimacy"? Today most people would define it as something more
than just the breakdown of formality into casual, easy relations,
marked by reasonable candor; they would instead define intimacy as being permitted to be unashamedly, confessionally
yourself, which would include spilling all the beans of your personal life, vast quantities of them, when the need to go on an
emotional spree arises.

Some friends need solace without being remotely in trouble.
Like the strict schoolteachers of an older day, these friends require perfect attendance. I have had a few such friends. My letting too long a time lapse between lunch or coffee dates was,
they somehow made clear, an injury to them. Irregularity in this
matter had the air of betrayal—better, of one's being responsible for jilting them. Whenever I was caught in such a friendship
—I usually ensnared myself through social cowardice, by not
drawing the line with sufficient clarity between friendliness and
friendship—I felt like nothing so much as a beautiful woman
who had committed herself to a homely and boring man whose
heart she felt it would be unconscionably cruel to break, though
God knows she longed to do so.

The problem with these friendships (if they really qualify for
the term) is that they invariably turned out to be one-sided. All

of them were with men who wished only to talk about themselves — their obsessions, wounds, grievances. It was as if the homely man, having arrived at the restaurant with the beautiful woman, wished only to gaze at himself in the restaurant mirror. Such people also had subtle ways of making plain their vulnerability. Should one turn them down, one risked adding to their already deep deposits of vulnerability and resentment.

Going along with such a friendship might seem feasible if one felt a backlog of previous kindnesses, acts of generosity, or altruism on the other person's part. But the reciprocity — even if based on acts of many years before — would have to have been there to make it seem just to put up with such subtle but quite real social tyranny. In the cases I have in mind, the backlog was never there.

Reciprocity is at the heart of friendship. This reciprocity is always of an inexact, probably immeasurable, doubtless best left unmeasured, nature. To ask for pure equivalence from a friend — I did this for you, therefore you must perform an act of precisely equal significance for me — is impossible, and shouldn't ever be required: to require it is an unfriendly act; it is to turn a friendship into a bartering relationship.

Yet this point isn't as clear as it might seem. Your introducing me to someone the meeting of whom greatly altered my life for the better may have had an importance to me well beyond the original effort on your own part. I, on the other hand, may have done many small favors for you, none of which touch this one in the magnitude of its importance, though it was casually intended on your part. In friendship, pure equivalence, or the balancing out of favors and kindnesses, probably cannot ever be achieved.

But somehow one recognizes equivalence in a friendship without having to have it spelled out or weighed up. Because you called to tell me that joke, I thought you ought to be alerted, by e-mail, to this excellent article in the current issue of the *Atlantic*. Because you took my wife and me to that splendid, reasonably priced Italian restaurant, I want to take you and your new lady friend to the seafood place my wife discovered through her cousin. Because you were helpful in giving my son advice about preparing for his interview at a stockbrokerage, advice that helped get him the job, I bought a necktie for you, thinking it would look great with your black cashmere blazer. Equivalence in friendship also covers less tangible but more important things: sympathy, for example, or patience, or generosity of spirit. Acceptance of oddity, or of social timidity, or of affection—all subtle and best never precisely formulated—also must be reciprocal.

Another of the obligations of friendship is accepting each other's weaknesses, flaws, limitations. "A friendly Eye is slow to see small Faults," writes Shakespeare in *Julius Caesar.* But sometimes the faults are not so small. Yet if the good feeling of friendship is strong, they can also be, if not quite overlooked, at least accepted as part of the deal of friendship. Making matters more complicated still, some of these—depression, self-absorption—may have been acquired later in life, long after the time when the friendship was initially formed. Perhaps everyone has friends, acquired when young, whom he or she wouldn't consider as possible friends if met today.

Everyone has known people whom, in order to like at all, one must like emphatically. I had such a friend—he died more than a decade ago—whose self-regard was so great, whose obsessions were so intense, and whose intensity itself was so off-putting to many people that the novelist Frank Conroy once said to me of him: "Do you know X? The guy is really sick." And so I suppose he might have seemed if one didn't happen to love him, which I did. My friend suffered the maladies of insomnia, paranoia, and megalomania, with the result that he spent many nights lying awake worrying about people taking power away from him that he didn't actually possess. His general tactlessness did not add luster to his personality. Yet this same man also had brilliance, integrity, loyalty, and courage, all of a high order. His virtues so outweighed his flaws that the former were not easily overlooked, but finally deserved to be, though on more than one occasion I myself had been stung as the victim of his tactlessness. I wish he were alive today to write a similar, single-paragraph character of me.

Whenever one uses the words "reciprocity" or "equivalence" in connection with friendship, one does well to assume the adjective "rough" before them. The reciprocity owed by a husband to a wife and a wife to a husband is much clearer, as is that between parents and children — some of it is even set out in law. But that among friends is subtler, more vague, yet no less crucial.

If I call this man or woman my friend, I owe him or her respect, candor, and tolerance, for starters. A friend should get the benefit of every doubt; as much slack as possible must be cut for him. What if a person you call friend, who has never acted but in a kindly and generous way toward you, is known in most of his other dealings to be the cause of misery in others — known as a snob, a bigot, an SOB generally? One has here a serious problem, the beginning approach to which is to ask why he has made an exception in never showing any of the unpleasant sides of himself to you. Weakness in a friend should be tolerated, but should character-crippling weakness of an uncivilized kind also be tolerated?

When I was nineteen I found myself in competition for the affection of a girl with another boy who was a friend — on the edge of being a close friend. Competitive in many ways — sports, gambling, literary reputation — I have never been competitive in the woman chase. I felt I hadn't the equipment — the powerful good looks — to win at this game; girls, then women, had almost to show they liked me first for me to become interested in them. But not this other fellow, who contended for everything. For reasons I cannot now recall, I seemed, in the phrase of the day, to be "beating him out" for the girl. So competitive was he, he would not speak to or even look at me. This was a weakness, I felt, that went to character. And while I still know him, now nearly half a century later, I have never allowed myself to grow any closer to him.

As I noted earlier, equality is neither a requirement nor an obligation of friendship, and in many friendships a strong and often irremediable inequality reigns quite happily. In his *Notebooks* Paul Valéry writes: "When Man grows up and grows old, his *friends-and-equals* is replaced by someone inferior, as though by a shadow. The system *Goethe-Schiller* gives way to the system *Goethe-Eckermann*. Valets as close friends, etc." None of us is Goethe, of course, but lots of people are willing to play one or another version of Eckermann, who agreed to perform the role of straight man, asking Goethe his views on everything, which the great writer was always ready to supply. One might befriend what we take to be a superior person for a variety of motives: to bask in the aura of his fame, to learn at his knee, to serve him out of a devotion that derives from genuine admiration, or various combinations of these and other reasons. He or she can also become, in effect, a trophy friend, someone to whom we can point to show our own rising status in the world.

In such a friendship the friend who is the trophy is under very little obligation other than to play the great man or woman, whereas the unequal or Eckermann friend is under the obligation to show continuing fascination with the genius, celebrity, power, or what have you of the ostensibly greater person. I was briefly in this type of friendship with the novelist Saul Bellow, who was twenty-one years older than I. Among the services I performed for him was to interview him, in the most genial way, for the *New York Times Book Review*. The friendship broke up for reasons I touch on briefly later in this book, but I knew I had become too closely identified as his friend when one day I had a call from a reporter from *Newsweek* asking if I could get him a picture of Bellow's fourth wife. The request made me feel less a friend than a valet.

Now I find that I may have become a trophy friend myself (third place, bronze) — emitting a rather soft, un-gem-like flame to which a small but insistent number of moths appear to be attracted. But there are obligations here, too, on the unequal side of the relationship. Even being flattered takes time: phone calls, coffee meetings, lunches. Sometimes these meetings involve the request for favors, for many of these people are would-be writers. Could I recommend an agent? Is there someone at *The New Yorker* to send a story to, and would it be all right to use my name? Would I be willing to read the first half of a novel in the works? New obligations form; more time is required to fulfill them.

Meanwhile, obligations to old friends and, on occasion, to their families, await, too often going unfulfilled. About many of these friends I feel, along with affection, lots of guilt. I have an older friend whose wife, who was easily his best friend, has died, leaving him inconsolably lonely. I call him once a week, exchange e-mails with him, send him books, go over to visit him occasionally, but not often enough. I like him a lot. But a better friend would do much more.

One of my friends is suffering depression, not clinical or chemically-caused depression, but what I think of as logical depression, which comes of discovering, too late to do much about it, that his life was mistakenly lived. I go to lunch with him when I can. But I can't bring myself to tell him that he is in danger of becoming seedy, needs to take better care of himself and his clothes, ought to pull up his socks, literally and figuratively. I can't tell him this because our friendship, though close, does not allow for me to offer him advice on how to live his life. I have abandoned him to the shrinks, who, charging him to listen to his woes, thus far haven't provided him all that much help. My behavior toward him here is not good enough — not for a real friend, it's not — and yet I don't know what to do.

Another friend, now dead, left a wife and daughter, who, following his death, have been going to pieces at a steady rate: making foolish financial deals, undertaking hopeless projects, falling into illness, lapsing into deeper and deeper neurosis. The daughter, who is the unsteadier of the two, once asked for help in a business venture. I turned her down. It's nuts to think I could help stop this juggernaut of sadness in my old friend's family, but my behavior here is defensible only in logic, and what is logically correct isn't always the same as what is morally correct, especially in friendship.

The questions that friendship raises in boldest relief are the fundamental ones: Whom do we live for? What are we on earth for, ourselves or others? Oughtn't altruism to have as strong a pull on us as egotism? Is love inevitably of less importance than self-love? La Rochefoucauld, the great anatomist of self-love and self-regard (for which he used the all-purpose term *amour-propre*) and its many cunning disguises, felt that friendship was "a mere traffic, wherein self-love always proposes to be a gainer." He also wrote that "we always love those who *admire* us; but we don't always love those whom we *admire.*" Behind many of the gestures of friendship La Rochefoucauld found business as usual — that is, everyone essentially out for himself.

But is this really so? The problem is that most of us are divided: we want to be kind, generous, reasonably sacrificing. It is only the bill for all this that comes to seem so steep. Torn, conflicted, riven, most people want to be good friends, which means fulfilling the obligations of friendship, but other obligations call out: to one's family, to one's work, to one's own requirements for selfish lazy contentment. What is to be done?

No one, I suspect, has a convincing answer to this vexing question. But the knowledge that no useful answer is available doesn't make it any less vexing, if only because one is faced with its consequences so frequently, especially with the passage of time. The older one's friends, perhaps the more insistently the question seems to be asked. A friend who has had Parkinson's disease for a number of years now has the torture of arthritis to go with it. She lives, alone, in New York. When my wife and I go to New York, we spend time with her, take her to dinner, to the movies. Over the phone we listen to her sad medical misadventures, condole with her about her pain. My wife, in fact, lifts most of the heavy weight here. But there isn't much else we can do. Of course, once again, it doesn't feel nearly enough.

I do not often get asked by friends to put them or their children up for jobs. But my view of friendship is not so pure that I feel one mustn't ask, or oughtn't to be asked, for such help, which is troubling only if the person one is asked to put forward clearly isn't qualified. When a person seems to me reasonably qualified, I do not think it an impingement on our friendship for me to do him or her a favor. I'm pleased that I can say, "Call so-and-so, and don't neglect to say that I suggested you do so." Or "Have her call me and we'll talk about it over lunch." As between whether this makes me feel important or I simply enjoy helping out, I believe you will know which interpretation I favor.

I have thus far in life been spared the obligation of having a friend ask me to do something seriously illegal on his behalf. I have a friend who, some years ago, was up for a government job that required a security clearance. When I was visited by a FBI man as part of her background check, he asked me if I knew anything controversial about her. I said that she sometimes took strong opinions in her writings on controversial questions and issues, neglecting to report that she was also living in a lesbian relationship, which she herself had never hidden. What if my friend had asked me, if queried on the matter, to deny that she was a lesbian? I would then have been presented with a very old dilemma — that between the individual and the state.

The novelist E. M. Forster, in 1938, just before England had gone to war against Germany, wrote, in an essay titled "What I Believe," "If I had to choose between betraying my country and betraying my friend, I hope I should have the guts to betray my country." Forster thought that the modern state was, by its very nature, opposed to personal relations, which he and his Bloomsbury friends, taking their cue from the English philosopher G. E. Moore, emphasized as being at the core of the good life sensitively lived. Forster has been accused of moral foolishness, for behind such a decision to betray one's country on behalf of one's friend is the need to take more careful account of the moral position of both friend and country. What if your friend were a Nazi or a Soviet spy intent on doing your country harm? Or a terrorist?

Aristotle, Cicero, and other ancient writers on friendship would contend that a true friend would never wish one to do anything that was not itself moral, noble, generous, virtuous. Cicero wrote that "the alliance of wicked men not only shouldn't be protected by a plea of friendship, but rather they should be visited with summary punishment of the severest kind, so that no one may think it permissible to follow even a friend when waging war against his own country." One wonders if Forster would have agreed. I suspect he wouldn't have.

The ancient, Aristotelian idea of friendship is that friends bring out the best in each other. Friends might have common backgrounds, similar affinities, like interests, but at its highest level friendship is about the formation and elevation of good character. Friendship that brings out corrupt or otherwise bad ends is, ipso facto, not true friendship. Real friends, good friends in the Aristotelian sense, confer benefits on one another; or as Aristotle put it, "It is more characteristic of a friend to do well by another than to be well done by, and to confer benefits is characteristic of the good man and of virtue." In fact, one of the reasons for having friends, Aristotle believed, was to have people for whom to do good. That is why even the perfectly happy man needed friends, and why without them he was incomplete.

In a true friendship, the question of living selfishly or selflessly doesn't come into play but is dissolved in the pure love of one friend for another. The not insignificant problem is to find a friend of high virtue, along with the allied problem of being such a friend oneself. I can confidently say, without the least false modesty, that, on either side, I myself do not qualify. I shall not answer for you.

# 8

❖

# *A Friendship Diary: Adulation, Stimulation, Obligation*

AFTER MUCH GRUMBLING about the exactions of friends in the preceding chapter, I decided, during the week of April 24–31, 2004, to keep a diary in which I recorded these exactions with some precision. What I discovered is that they weren't, in fact, all that exacting. Whether this week turned out to be exceptional in the lightness of its meetings and distractions, I can't be sure. Certainly it was lighter than many weeks I can recall in which I had three or four lunch dates, an equal number of meetings for coffee, and a night or two out for dinner during the middle of the week.

For many people, the number of such get-togethers with friends as I have described in the previous sentence would, I realize, be thought a fairly light social load and the notion of a lunch or evening spent alone the social equivalent of a punishment. I'm not sure how this came about, but I have become the sort of man who looks at his calendar at the beginning of the week and when he finds very few set meetings or appointments says to himself, "Ah, looks like a good week."

Once, when I was complaining of the heavy traffic I had in friends at all levels, someone (a friend, naturally) asked me what I got out of all these meetings. "Stimulation," I said. "Maybe adulation, too," he suggested, a more knowing tone in his voice than I liked. All writers are pigs for praise, and, as a writer, my own appetite in this line, to put it gently, is not puny. Viewing my weeklong diary, I note that a large number of my calls, e-mails, and meetings are with former students and with people I have come to know through their once offering a good opinion of my writing. Is a prerequisite of becoming my friend admiration for my writing? Has my vanity already reached this pathetic stage?

On the other side, it probably ought to be said that most friendships don't begin with open avowals of admiration for the other party's skill, as so many of mine have. The following postcard seems more than a bit improbable: "I've admired your dentistry for years, and I wonder if you are free one afternoon to meet me for coffee?" Nor do dentists typically have people ask them, "Can you tell me what you think about this filling I've just made? Do I have any talent?" But people don't mind writing or saying such things to writers, sometimes with the added minor request that they would be especially pleased if the writer would agree to sign one of his books for them. If the writer is someone in my condition — not used to heavy commercial success, grateful that someone has actually paid $25 or so for one of his books, touched that the person was kind enough to call or send a note afterward to say that his writing gave much pleasure — he would have to be unusually cold, or firmly disciplined, to say, "Whaddya, kiddin' me? No way, no, absolutely not, no chance, Lance. Screw off." Certainly he is not going to do so if the person requesting the meeting seems sane and intelligent (and that they must be both if they think well of his writing goes almost without saying).

I am extremely lucky in apparently having some quality in my writing that at least a little resembles that possessed by the writer described in *The Catcher in the Rye,* who, after you read him, Holden Caulfield tells us, you wish to call him on the phone. Perhaps this is owing to my being one of those writers who do not bring his readers shocking news from unexplored worlds but instead often formulate thoughts that they themselves hold, if inchoately. Whatever the reason, I have always felt myself fortunate in my readers; the people who have written to me about my writing have been overwhelmingly kind and tactful, almost never pushy, dreary, or *chutzpadik* in any way. When they have requested a meeting, these meetings, with the rare exceptions of people wishing to talk exclusively about themselves, have been enjoyable, often informative, and generally pleasing.

Edward Shils used to say that there were four modes of education available in modern societies: schools, serious periodicals, new and used bookshops, and the intelligent conversation of friends. And one of these modes will become more important than the others at a particular stage of a person's life. When Edward was alive, the conversation of friends, especially with him but also with the people he introduced me to, many international scholars among them, was perhaps of primary importance. He had only to speak for me to learn new factual information, a comic possibility, or a significant connection that had hitherto not occurred to me: the writer Camille Paglia, I only the other day recall his saying, "was much more intelligent than her ideas." No friend I have had was so stimulating, nor do I expect another ever to be, as my friend Edward.

Yet stimulation I do get from my various friends, from some of course more than others. Older friends, though for obvious reasons diminishing in number, often fill me in on bits of information known only before my time: Dr. Loyal Davis, Nancy Reagan's stepfather, I recently learned from a friend in his late eighties, was known in Chicago as a rabid anti-Semite. Others have pointed out the former locations around town of once infamous speakeasies and bordellos. I have superior discussions, at roughly three-month intervals, about baseball and other matters, with a hematologist who first wrote to me about an essay I published in *The New Yorker* on the subject of bypass surgery, which, like me, he had also undergone. With old friends, with whom I go back to high school, I enjoy keeping up on the fates of our various classmates. Not long ago, I reestablished contact with a University of Chicago roommate whom I hadn't seen in more than forty years, and enjoyed myself a lot in his company. Friends may not lead me onto the path of virtue, as Aristotle and Cicero thought the best of friends ought to do, but the more lively among them keep me interested and amused — not small things — for which I am grateful.

For some friends I feel chiefly a sense of obligation. Not that there is anything wrong with that. Older friends lose husbands or wives, get ill, can become depressed, live more and more in the past, cease listening. And the same thing can happen to one-self, who may one day require the tolerance of younger friends. I'm reminded here of a then-young gay man I knew who once told me that he used sometimes to give himself to an older man in the baths, in the hope that, as he phrased it, "some beautiful young thing such as I now am will give himself to me when I'm an old guy." That struck me at the time as a reasonable proposi-tion, and it still does.

It is possible, of course, to derive both adulation and stimula-tion from a friendship and yet also feel a strong sense of obliga-tion, if only to repay the pleasure of the gifts of the first two qualities. At its heart, friendship is about unreckonable reci-procity, incalculable equivalence.

Here is my friendship diary:

### Saturday, April 24

1. Wrote a (lying) e-mail to LF, telling him I could not meet him in Evanston anytime next weekend when he will be in Chicago. I like him but not well enough to cut into my weekend by driving downtown to join him for lunch.

2. On morning walk back from Jewel supermarket, ran into HW; stopped at Dempster Street Starbucks for forty-five min-utes of schmooze. I know HW from high school days — he is a couple of years younger than I — and find him more attractive as we grow older. We go out roughly once a year with our wives; all four of us get on well. He has drawn bad health cards in life: has already had two bypass surgeries and a few years ago was found to be diabetic. He senses that he is unlikely to be as long-lived as everyone else now hopes to be: most of us will, unreal-istically, feel cheated if we don't get to eighty-five or more. He has a more acute sense than most that the game could be up at any moment, which, without interfering with his good humor, has given it a nice gallows quality.

3. Drove out to Glencoe to pick up MR; drove to Beinlich's

for old-fashioned hamburger lunch with his son, daughter-in-law, and two grandsons. MR's son, who has become very authoritative, did most of the talking. Recall Mikhail Chilewich, a serious patron of Jewish charities, saying to me upon meeting me: "I'm much older than you, have less long to live, therefore I'll do most of the talking." MR, who is in his late eighties, could have, but did not play the Chilewich card.

4. Stopped to order two pair of khaki trousers from Irwin Lipps at Huntley's, his shop in Plaza del Lago. Told story of the three men imagining what others might say when standing over their coffins to Rusty, the young salesman there, who requested a joke. Irwin, who is sixty-three, is someone I much like, a friend of many years, yet one of the far middle distance. One bad year he had a heart attack, a cancer surgery, and a divorce — a trifecta of *tsouris*. We have never met outside his shop — never discussed meeting for lunch or a dinner. Nor are there any plans for us to do so. This arrangement seems OK for both of us.

5. Drove B [my wife] downtown to pick up her ceramics pieces at her teacher-friend Vanessa S's studio in the Fine Arts Bldg. Drove Vanessa to the gallery to pick up a work of her own, thence back to the Fine Arts Bldg., thence home. B is more tender-, which is to say good-, hearted than I. She goes much further out of her way for people; has an especially large sympathy for people who are alone in the world.

6. Wrote an e-mail to thank MR for flowers he sent home for B after our lunch.

7. Received an e-mail from CW, remarking on my George Steiner piece, telling me further Steiner anecdotes, suggesting a meeting in the summer. I've met him once before; the meeting was agreeable enough, but am not sure that I require another, even though I think him highly intelligent and regard him as one of the good guys: a man who in print has established his seriousness about great writing.

### Sunday, April 25

1. Wrote an e-mail to CK, to compliment him on, and remark upon, his piece on Karl Joachim Weintraub, an old teacher of mine and (much later) his at the University of Chicago. Funny

one-way arrangement here; I've sent him things I've written which he never comments on. I always comment on things he sends me. Think I shall desist from commenting on future compositions of his; see if he takes my point.

2. E-mails from RG (longish, about attending a party, feeling more reconciled to his son's suicide) and LJ (shortish, about his brother's remembering their father buying George Mashbitz suits [Mashbitz was a high-end Chicago tailor whose name occurs in a short story of mine]).

3. Answered jokey e-mail from TC. Another literary one-way-street man who sends me his stuff to read and praise; never remarks on mine. Haven't seen him for fifteen years. Still, I like him.

4. AG calls, telling me about his new cable hookup and suggesting a Czech film B and I might want to see. Small but pure altruistic gesture.

5. I write to ER, my editor at Oxford University Press, *shnorring* a new biography of Mendelssohn. ER is someone I like without knowing her very well. Relationships with editors, especially book editors, are odd, not least because they, the editors, tend to move on and out of one's ken. I liked LW, then at Houghton Mifflin, quite a bit; his was a vaguely therapeutic style. He told me some mildly intimate things. He moved on to Farrar, Straus and Giroux and I haven't heard from him since. Probably shan't, unless he has a project to propose or I happen to run into him in a restaurant or on the streets of New York. Nothing wrong with this; it is merely the way it is. I've lost touch with most of my past book editors, with one exception, all of whom I've liked and spoken with in the same quasi-intimate way. No business like lit business, I guess.

6. Received e-mail (on Santayana and the Tragic Sense) from RG. He and I have never met — a retired college teacher, he lives in a small town in South Carolina — and, I suspect, never will meet. He reads poetry with great intensity and deep enjoyment. He lapses into dark views, which he often reports to me. My job then is to help him out of his *shlunk* by instructing him to calm down and stay on the job. He doesn't seem to resent my doing so.

## Monday, April 26

1. Answered e-mail from RM, a former student, probably my best student, whom I much like and whose career I will do anything I can to promote. Of all my former students, he is the one whom I feel is closest to a contemporary, though I'm more than thirty years older. He has very high intellectual standards. I sometimes worry that they might be impossibly high. Too high standards, never permitted any slack, is one of the surest ways I know to a sad life.

2. E-mails from EH, a former student (now nearing forty) with whom I have an amiable, mostly jokey relationship. We always mention getting together for lunch or a Cubs game, but almost never do. We actually don't need regular meetings to be reminded of our inherent good feeling for each other. A bachelor, he once told me that he couldn't spend much time with a woman who didn't deeply appreciate irony. A bachelor he may well long remain.

3. Visit from PF, ostensibly for me to sign a book of mine she is planning to give as a gift. Half-hour stay, during which we talked about her thirteen-year-old son and my fourteen-year-old granddaughter. PF is a woman of astounding energy and a great propensity for doing good, which she really does. She went on a little tirade about George W. Bush. I let her get it out of her system.

4. Long call from GW; much talk about his twenty-one-year-old son, with whom I spent a few hours and who is depressed because he has high cultural aspirations without being able to do anything to establish his cultural bona fides. At his age, how could he? I've met with the kid, who is serious. His father is in no position to understand quite why the boy is unhappy. I'm in a position to understand but was able to do nothing to assuage it. One's obligations extend beyond one's friends to the children of one's friends. Ah, friendship! Ah, humanity! Ah, screw it!

5. Longer call from ST; there goes the morning. He and I generally engage in literary talk, much of it gossip division. We did again today—much to my wastrel's pleasure.

6. Lunch with WP, who seemed less depressed, rather more responsive, than usual. Was able to get him to tell me that he is

seeing a shrink. He has what I believe is a late-life crisis, in which his regrets heavily outweigh his achievements. If one is a thoughtful person, as WP is, pharmacology can provide relief, can lighten the load of sadness, but is finally not all that much in the way of help. Even friends who love him, as I do, can't do much, except tell him not to lose the time that is left to him in sadness and further regret. And I don't even do this, lest I offend him by the obviousness of such advice.

7. E-mail from LJ, who has done an interview with me that, my guess is, he is going to be unable to place.

8. Letter from CP: standard complaints about the world going to hell, intellectual and social standards falling, led by the ignorant young. Hard to know what to say in response to this. CP heading toward eighty; arguing the pointlessness of his views with him itself seems pointless. Occurs to me that when older people say the world is going to hell what they really mean to say is how good can it be when I shall soon no longer be in it. I write back, ignoring his complaints, tell him what I've been reading that he might want to look into.

9. RG yet again. He generally sends me at least one e-mail a day, sometimes three or four. I try to answer them all, providing laconic answers, because I have limited time.

## Tuesday, April 27

1. Phone call — B took it — from a man named Tony Kelly, reporting that he and I "have friends in common." He didn't say who; promised (threatened?) to call back.

2. A call from SR, a woman from my old neighborhood [West Rogers Park], though eight or so years younger than I, and a reader of mine, now living in Marin County. Wants to meet for coffee. I may have suggested it in an earlier exchange of e-mails, thinking she wouldn't follow through. But now she has.

3. A joke from SS about grandchildren. I've never met him. He is a reader of mine, in *Commentary* and elsewhere. A well-to-do lawyer, he once wanted me to write a screenplay about a wealthy man who faked a military record so that he might be buried in Arlington Cemetery. The project, like most film projects, never came off.

4. RG e-mail, then yet another.

5. I call CN, B's and my friend from *Britannica* days, about Cubs tickets. B takes her to a Cubs game every year.

6. KT, whom I called earlier to talk about my meeting with WP, returned my call, which I missed.

7. Met MB, who claims me as a mentor of sorts, though I was never her teacher, at Osco pharmacy; we walked back together to my apartment talking about her novel, for which I have suggested an agent. I like her a lot and want her to succeed.

8. MB afterward sent me an e-mail saying that Lourdes Lopez, the literary agent, with whom I had put her in touch, has received the revisions to her ms and is ready to send it off to Penguin/Viking.

## Wednesday, April 28

1. Returned e-mail to NG, a reader and professional photographer who went to the University of Chicago and whom I also met, once, for coffee and schmooze: we spent a pleasant two hours but am not sure I require more.

2. Sent postcard to DC, a former student, now perhaps fifty, congratulating him on the birth of a son.

3. E-mails on my *WSJ* piece on the Cheerful Conservative from Denis Dutton, of artsandlettersdaily.com, and AG.

4. Sent letter with three dollars included to Joe Dekin, my former student Elaine's seven-year-old son. His father, Tim, who taught at Northwestern when I was there and whom I much liked, died a few years ago. The sadness of kids who do not grow up with both their parents is one I shall never get used to.

5. Exchanged e-mails with DW, a former student, very smart and talented, and someone I like a great deal.

6. Call on voice mail from EM, who invites B and me to dinner with her and her husband. I've met her for coffee a few times. She mostly talks about herself and her brilliant career, searches for ways I might help her find a commercial publisher for her academic books. Decide not to return the call.

7. Note to Phil Kaufman, the movie director, with whom I went to high school and, afterward, to the University of Chicago, consoling him for the merciless reviews his new movie, *Twisted,* has received from critics. The best I could offer in the way of consolation was to inform him of my belief in the low

quality of movie critics, adding that no one should devote his life to forming opinions about the achievements of other people — which is to say that being a full-time movie critic probably isn't such a hot idea if one wishes to be a serious person. Not much consolation provided here, I suspect.

8. Received copy of his new book about his father and the New Deal heritage with a nice inscription from MJ. Wrote to thank him.

9. Call from not Tony but now Anthony Kelly, announcing himself as friend of friends: Bob McCollough and Dick Gosswiller, whom I knew and liked forty-four years ago. He told me that Bob McC, a splendid photographer and a very genial man, is long dead.

10. Call from NB, reporting to me on an Old Boys meeting at Briarwood Country Club — a meeting that I shall not attend. Have lost my taste — permanently? — for talking about the days of our youth. Have by now heard most of these stories seven and eight times. I'd rather have NB's report on the meeting, which he will eventually give me, than spend the four or so hours attending it.

11. Exchange of e-mails (with not very good joke) from TS, another reader, a nice man, a conservative who believes the sky is falling. I tell him to lay off all those Chicken Little books he reads that predict the decline and death of everything good.

12. Call from Bonnie Nims, the widow of John Frederick Nims; set up lunch meeting on May 7. Bonnie is someone B and I see twice, perhaps three times a year, another middle-distance friend, but someone who always seems to us, especially after her husband's death, and despite her many health problems, without the least touch of self-pity and therefore quite gallant.

13. Possible lunch meeting, suggested through e-mail, with JB, who is coming to Chicago. I have come to know him through my close friend GF. (One of the side-benefit gifts of friendship is, of course, friends introducing one to other friends.) JB is a former teacher and dean at Indiana University at Indianapolis and a man with cosmopolitan tastes in literature and art. He is attracted to the dark in art while being entirely cheerful in life. We fill each other in on reading or movies the other doesn't know about, and laugh about the pretentiousness of academics, which is always in good supply.

14. Phone call from SR, setting up coffee date for tomorrow.

15. Letter from CG, a reader and a very nice woman, asking for a picture from me for the Skokie Public Library, where she has worked, without a degree in library science, for many years. She is a good and intelligent person and a passionate reader. I find it difficult to say no to her about anything.

### Thursday, April 29

1. Answered JB, telling him I can't make lunch next week.

2. E-mail from AG, announcing his new e-mail address.

3. E-mail from BM, a fairly recent widower and a screenwriter who lives in Los Angeles, about my *WSJ* piece, which I answered. He is someone I knew only glancingly during college years, but have come to like more and more. Years go by during which we don't see each other. He can be lugubrious, but manages to be humorous even about his own lugubriousity.

4. Answered e-mails from MR, KW (director of the Washington office of the Hudson Institute), SF (former student, an East Indian brought up in Indiana, who once told me that he and his pals used to play a game called Who's Your Favorite Hoosier?), RP, and AK.

5. An e-mail from EML, remarking on my *WSJ* piece and inviting B and me to her and her husband's fiftieth anniversary party in San Francisco, which I'm fairly certain we shall not attend.

6. E-mail exchange with SW, an oncologist at Northwestern and a friend of (perhaps) four years duration, about going to a Cubs-Giants game on May 20.

7. E-mail exchange with DL, librarian at Western Michigan, about my *WSJ* piece. I've never met him; perhaps never shall. Our friendship is entirely on-line.

8. E-mails to BM and RG.

9. Ninety-minute coffee with SR, who is in town for a Boone School reunion and has written to me about my books. A lively person, not shy about talking about herself. Very energetic. Another woman alone.

10. Talked with LC and MC about dinner reservation for tomorrow night, at Erwin's. MC is our family lawyer, and has become a friend over the years.

### Friday, April 30

1. E-mails this A.M. to DZ, with whom I am back in touch after many decades out of touch, RG, and KW.

2. E-mail to PL, checking on his troubles. He married late and has had three daughters with a much younger woman and is now undergoing a difficult and complicated divorce. He does not have an excessive amount of money.

3. Phone call from MJ, thanking me for e-mail, filling me in on the critical success of his book, suggesting a meeting when next I am in New York — a meeting that will probably not take place.

4. B's and my old friend (from grammar school days) CP here after her and B's lunch together. Drove her home before we met the Cs for dinner at Erwin's. Much admire CP's courage in living uncomplainingly with multiple sclerosis. B's good heart once again to the fore, wonderfully thoughtful about her friend.

5. Medical appointment with JR, my gastroenterologist, who has become a middle-distance friend. He e-mails me vast number of jokes. Much laughter during appointment. He sends me home with a huge bag of Prevacid samples.

6. Dinner with LC and MC. Badgering putdown humor resides — playful teasing, MC's specialty. I give as good as I get, I do believe, and no one comes out the worse for it.

7. E-mail from SLN, whom I meet every six weeks or so for coffee and pleasing chatty talks about our common past as kids, imploring me to come to Boone School reunion, which I have no intention of doing. We set up a coffee meeting for next week, at ten, before she goes off to work.

As I read over these diary entries, I note the fairly large amount of e-mail communication, which I much like, for it is more sparing of time than long phone conversations, for which I have a weakness. I note, too, the small number of lunches during this week (just two); Henry James called social lunches "those matutinal monsters" for the way they destroyed his afternoons. For all that this weeklong diary may not be completely representative of my social life, it does, I think, give some notion of the mixture of demands, delights, and complications that a mildly gregarious man in his sixties encounters from and with friends over the course of seven days. The unanswered question is, what would I feel if no one called, wrote, sent e-mail, or wanted to meet for lunch, dinner, or coffee? Pause for silence here, after which, in a gruff voice-over, we hear: "Enough complaining. Shut up and finish your biscotti!"

# 9

❖

# *Pity Is at the Bottom*
# *of Women*

ACCORDING TO THE RECEIVED opinion of the day, women are better at friendship than are men. They are now thought better because, the feeling is, they are less nervous about the commitments required by friendship, less edgy and anxious about opening themselves up to the wide-ranging emotions of friendship. Women, one such study by a woman has it, "have the opportunity to acknowledge our need for other women as well as our need for recognition and acceptance of our autonomous selves." This is so — again I'm reporting the received opinion — because they are less competitive, which means less rivalrous, than men. They are also more easily given to intimacy and are thought to rush less quickly to judgment, which can put a terrible crimp in friendship. "Judgmental" has, in our day, become a pejorative word and distinctly not a good thing to be.

For centuries, women were not even considered worthy of membership in the realm of friendship. (Recall Montaigne on the subject.) Women could be queens or the secret powers behind men who ruled — in ancient Sparta women were thought to be a bold force and in the Roman Empire they were often that, without doubt — and there were among aristocratic women of later times (Madame de Staël and Madame Récamier,

in the early nineteenth century, for notable example) friendships of great depth of feeling. But in the classical discussions of
friendship, women were by and large excluded.

All this changed, if slowly, with first the political emancipation and then the social and psychological emancipation of
women that followed therefrom. Not that women hadn't always
befriended one another through the ages. But women in groups
were not studied; nor were their friendships taken seriously except in novels. Female friendship is a strong element in Jane
Austen, but marriage always provided the central drama. Men
have travels and adventures, an old saying had it, and women
have lovers and husbands. The real meaning behind the saying
is that the true lives of women were lived through their men —
that outside their men, and later their children and family life,
they didn't quite exist.

No one would any longer maintain this is so. Although
equality of condition is not everywhere the case, many — perhaps most — women, in the West anyway, may now be said to
lead lives at least partially independent of men and, if they wish,
of their own families. Women, the English novelist Sue Limb
writes in her essay "Female Friendship," "are stronger as indi-
viduals, less dependent on men for our sense of ourselves, and
emancipated from and hostile to many brutal and competitive
values which have deformed male-dominated society." And at
the center of these women's lives is, along with work, friendships with other women.

But how are these friendships different from friendships
among men? According to most women, they are much, even
radically, different. A great many women, including married
women, are quick to report that their female friendships are
their main support in life. The title *I Know Just What You
Mean*, a book about female friendship by the columnist Ellen
Goodman and the novelist Patricia O'Brien, captures, especially that word *Just*, something of the ready rapport women
are felt to share that is usually unavailable to men. Surveys have
been taken in which many men claim that their wives are their
best friends, while these same wives claim their best friends are
in fact other women.

The standard complaint in these cases, though different in its details, usually comes under the general heading of male insensitivity to female interests. "The average woman knows 275 colors — men know 8" is a line from a poem called "Men Say Brown," by Henry M. Seiden, which makes a nice point about what can sometimes seem the fundamental differences between men and women. Women not only — and quite naturally — find more common interests among other women, but they enjoy an easier candor on subjects of both significance and intimacy with other women. I don't know how high the truth quotient for the television program *Sex and the City* is, but a similar program about men being utterly candid with one another on their personal relationships is unthinkable.

Friendships among women can differ according to country and social class, but, to cite Sue Limb again, at the heart of most female friendships is "a mixture of sympathy and instruction: of a loving heart and a shrewd eye." Among themselves women are capable of "a careless honesty," a willingness to expose their vulnerability that does not come naturally, if ever, to men. Envy, jealousy, impatience, and anger can play their divisive roles in many female friendships, to be sure, but at the center one feels the nature of friendship among women is somehow lighter, but also deeper, and often more genuinely disinterested because less rivalrous.

Women seem greater suckers than men for the therapy centers, encounter groups, and other such enterprises that continue to flourish in America. (These have long since caught on with men, too, some of whom meet in what are essentially extended therapy groups over full weekends, where they talk about doubts connected with their identity, their masculinity, their vulnerabilities, and then — shudder — they hug a lot.) But women among themselves also seem to be able to shoot straighter with one another than do men. A woman can usually tell another woman that her choice of the man she is going with is wrong, a big mistake. A man can almost never tell another man that he is with the wrong woman without incurring genuine anger: "What's it your freakin' business, shmuckowitz!"

Men have a greater sense of La Rochefoucauld's *amour-*

*propre,* with all the phrase suggests of an easily bruised ego. This sense is the principal mechanism by which men are able to practice self-deception, sometimes to the point of making rollicking jackasses of themselves. Women are not completely without *amour-propre,* but they do not generally seem to possess it to the high comic power that men frequently do: most comedy, as the eighteenth-century dramatists knew, begins with exaggerated claims to dignity, often a masculine specialty.

Women are also, I believe, less given to fantasy than are men. While many men believe that they had—even late in life continue to have—it in them to be great athletes, lovers, and business geniuses, and are often prepared to suggest as much in conversation with other men, woman are not as prone to empty bragging or recounting old victories in the sack or on the playing fields of business. Women seem less status-minded, at least in friendships, than do men; they can more easily be comfortable with friends who have much less or more money than they. Most women are also able to confide in one another without great difficulty. (Men are often made nervous by these confidences, and especially prefer not to dwell on their own inadequacies.) One sociological study showed that men often confide more easily in women than they do in other men.

The most widely accepted received opinion on this subject is that intimacy is easier for women than it is for men, and that this is particularly so among small groups of women. Yet one wonders if this is really true. The English novelist Arnold Bennett, in his *Journal* (for May 25, 1908), remarks: "It occurred to me, for the first time I do believe, that women, when very intimate, have coolnesses and difficulties just as men do and perhaps more . . . I can see the origin of my error, dimly; it has something to do with the idea of women solidifying themselves together in a little group as distinguished from the whole male sex, of them understanding each other so much better than any man could understand them, that they understand and sympathize with each other to absolute perfection. Curious misconception, but natural." In his *Notebooks* Paul Valéry writes: "We can be truly intimate only with people having our own standard of *discretion.*" This sounds right to me. A woman who talks in intricate detail about her sex life is unlikely to be warmly welcomed by a woman who thinks this a wholly private matter.

A passage from E. M. Forster's *Howards End* comes closer, I feel, to the truth of the matter of why women are more sympathetic than men to a wider range of confidences from their friends, male and female. "Pity, if I may generalize, is at the bottom of woman." Forster writes. "When men like us, it is for our better qualities, and however tender their liking, we dare not be unworthy of it, or they will quietly let us go. But unworthiness stimulates woman. It brings out her deeper nature, for good or for evil." A subtle passage, this, which I take to mean that women — not all, of course, but women in the main — are more sympathetic to failure than are men.

I have a friend, a woman fifteen or so years younger than I, a writer and true nonconformist in her manner of dress, expression, interests. Not long ago she told me that she has a friend with a towering IQ who appears to have an accompanying personal difficulty for every point of IQ he possesses. He is, according to her account, very odd-looking, gay but with no known sex life, unable to make a living, filled with phobias, still squatting in the home of his now aged parents. And yet my friend found something in him that I am reasonably certain I never would. She has stayed in touch with him — he is, she reports, exceptionally witty — encouraged him to do something with his astounding mathematical ability, pushed him out into the world in a gentle way. She has done all this without motive. She is herself married but childless, and so perhaps this man, strange duck that he is, brought out her maternal instincts. Whether this is so I do not pretend to know. I do know that no man would have done for him what she has. A perfect illustration, or so it seems to me, of Forster's point that "pity is at the bottom of woman."

I recently heard, from a man, a story about his wife and two other women, all in their fifties, visiting their former college roommate, who was in the last weeks of a losing bout with cancer. All had traveled from distant points to Wisconsin, where she lived, to say a final goodbye. The four women were comfortable in this situation, and the woman who was dying had somehow arranged to make the visit seem a cheering and far from sad occasion. The man who told me the story remarked that seeing the four old friends together was so heartening that he took the three husbands of these women out to shoot pool so that the women might have more time alone together. Difficult, I think, to imagine four male friends bringing off something as impressive as this.

Men are less good at accepting death. A man does not wish to hear about another man's fears, unpleasant secrets, deep disappointments — unless, perhaps, he is paid to do so as a psychotherapist. Not that women necessarily are eager to hear about these things either, but they do not automatically declare them out of bounds, as men tend to do. Women may or may not be able to handle intimacy more easily than men — some would argue that they are also on more intimate terms with their own bodies, beginning with the rude introduction to the intimacy of anatomy that they experience as young girls by way of menstruation — but they do not seem, like men, to have been trained to be put off by it.

Friendships among women are of course no less various than those among men; the categories of such friendships no fewer. There are friendships between girls, adolescent girls, married women, single women. (Oddly and interestingly, everyone seems to agree that adolescent girl friendships never work well in threesomes; two of the trio will always find a way to side against the third, in a manner that is certain to hurt her. A number of recent novels have taken up this subject.) The category "single women" breaks down further, into never-married women, divorced women, women living in unmarried sexual relationships (with men or with other women), widows, lesbians. Like men, women ask different things of friendship at different stages of their lives: the kinds of friendships women have in their twenties figure to be quite different from those they have in their sixties or seventies.

Even now, despite all the talk of the breakdown of the patriarchal system in which men clearly were dominant, the rise of feminism, and the wider acceptance of male and female homo-sexuality, the norm in Western life still is the married heterosex-ual couple. This remains true even when marriage in the United States is down to 56 percent for adults, with only 26 percent of Americans living in a household with children. It remains true even when more women are working, have a stronger sense of themselves apart from men, and have a vastly wider range of so-cial and economic opportunities. Yet, for all this, women are still more socially hostage to men than men to women — that is, in a strong sense their relations to men continue to define them in a way that isn't true of most men's relations to women. (Per-haps this so because women, however liberated their views, know that they are responsible for maintaining the home and setting its standard of comfort and amenities.)

The old-fashioned word "spinster," for example, always im-plied an older woman unable to find a man. An older, lifelong bachelor, on the other hand, was more likely to have been thought to have chosen his fate of solitariness. In the same vein, a woman who has married a successful and good man is often viewed as having a successful life, while a man who has married a highly intelligent and good-hearted woman is merely thought lucky: a woman's whole life, that is, may still be judged on her marriage, a man's rarely so.

In an age of high divorce rates, strong feminism, of open and (probably) increasing lesbianism, the conjugal role still seems central for women. Because of this, marital status often provides an organizing principle for female friendships. A mar-ried woman in her forties or older is unlikely to have a majority of women friends who have never married. Marriage also gives women what one might call a core curriculum of conversation subjects: raising children, real estate, cooking, husbands (not excluding the dreariness of husbands).

Social class can provide another organizing principle of fe-male friendship: in a more class-conscious country such as Eng-land, not many solidly middle- or upper-middle-class women are likely to have working-class friends. In America, a woman can fall from her upper-middle-class status and still retain her upper-middle-class friends. The best friend of a woman who is a friend of mine, for example, is a waitress in an Italian restaurant. My friend has told me that, among the attractions she finds in this dear friend is that she has a greater grip on the reality of the workaday world, herself being dab in the center of it.

Friendships among women are frequently thought to supply what husbands or male lovers cannot or do not know how to supply: an attentive audience, sympathy for common problems (female health and child-rearing problems among them), talk about the pleasures of clothes or shopping, detached humor about the flaws of men. The husband behind his newspaper at the breakfast table not listening to his wife has been a stock figure in *New Yorker* cartoons for decades. Sometimes women help one another out through babysitting; sometimes they enjoy the simple pleasures of association (with no added sense of obligation entailed); sometimes they do share intimacy of a kind that is unavailable in their relations with their husbands.

Some men feel a certain jealousy for their wives' or lovers' friends, sensing that the latter are providing them with things that they don't. (They are probably right, if not to feel jealous, then at least envious, owing to their own inability to supply these things.) They may also sense that their wives or lovers, meeting with women friends, are laughing at them—at their pretensions, their coarseness, their less than dazzling sexual performance. (They may be right again.) Men seem to want to dominate women in ways that women don't usually care to dominate them. Perhaps it's that old masculine *amour-propre* once again raising its humorless head: "You Jane, Tarzan's woman." Jane, it has now become abundantly clear, doesn't agree.

Women, too, may be intrinsically more sociable than men. They seem better at giving parties, and at organizing the parties they do give: hostesses almost always seem better at the social task than hosts. They are willing to put more time and thought into seating, menu, guest list, and other items that make for greater social comfort. A strong feminist might dismiss this by saying that all such details are of a triviality beneath the seriousness of men and of intelligent women. Or, again, the objection might be that it's simply a function of socialization—that girls are taught to care about these things and boys are not. I don't happen to think these objections hold up. Skills of an important kind—they are called graciousness and hospitality—are involved. Besides, as anyone who has a nodding acquaintance with French intellectual history knows, women organized and ran the great salons of the seventeenth and eighteenth centuries and were key figures in the cultural life of France. And not only in France. Jonathan Swift felt that the "degeneracy of conversation [in his day] hath been owing, among other causes, to the custom arisen, for some time past, of excluding women from any share in our society." A sense of social consideration, a feeling for sociability, of making friends comfortable, is in question, and such skills aren't always, or even usually, available to men, which is a deficiency.

This carries over into the differences in conversational style between men and women. Women tend to be calmer, cooler, viewing conversation less as a competition than as a means of drawing one another out. In *The Sex Game,* the sociologist Jessie Bernard attempts to distinguish between the way men and women go at conversation. Men, she found, were more competitive in conversation, seeing it as one more battlefield from which to emerge with the victory of seeming more analytical, reasonable, smarter than one's interlocutor. Conversation, for men, often becomes debate by other means, with points awarded for logic, reasoning, unassailable positions, firm conclusions.

If I may drop a name here (it's no longer as good a name, alas, as it once was), many years ago the playwright Lillian Hellman told me that the literary critic Edmund Wilson was two different persons, depending on whether he was talking to a man or a woman. If Wilson was talking to a man, he would play the schoolyard bully, who had to show that no one knew more about any subject under discussion than he; apparently he had to knock the other man down intellectually. But if he was talking to a woman, he could be fatherly, avuncular, kind, on some occasions gently seductive.

Aligned with their general competitiveness in conversation, some men specialize in being aggressive in conversational style.

One can think of women with such a style—Dorothy Parker, Bette Midler, Alice Roosevelt Longworth—but these are exceptions that prove the rule of women behaving differently. For certain men, aggressiveness in conversation is a set style. The putdown, the relentless one-upmanship, the ironic thrust, these are all familiar male conversational ploys. I have a number of male friendships in which this mock aggressiveness is the chief note. In handling a real estate closing for me, my lawyer, who is also a friend, was asked by the seller's agent, who happened to be a reader of mine, if he had known me long: "Oh," he replied, "I knew him when he was still virile." Hard to imagine two women in similar banter: "I knew her when she was still fertile (sexy, beautiful, elegant)." Not likely.

Jessie Bernard writes of women using conversation for "stroking," by which she means making the other person feel secure, well disposed, good about him- or herself. Unless they happen to be selling something, many men don't see it that way, preferring to come away from lots of conversations feeling, to a greater or lesser extent, better about *themselves*. Men, Professor Bernard writes, are more at home with language in its "instrumental," or task-doing function; women with language in its "expressive," or less direct, sometimes purely artistic, function.

The stereotype of the chatterbox woman notwithstanding, my sense is that women are probably better, if only because more patient, listeners. (This despite the joke about the boy who returns home to tell his mother that he is playing a Jewish husband in his school play, causing her to call the teacher to demand a speaking part for her son.) Men often seem eager to get talk over with—to get, in the cant phrase, to the bottom line. The novelist John O'Hara remarked that no woman who graduated from high school ever used the phrase "half a buck"; I find it difficult to imagine any woman today saying, "So what's the bottom line here?"—at least not in a social setting.

As I grow older, I find fewer and fewer men who truly listen to one another. Usually they more or less politely wait for the next man to cease talking so that they can have their go. They are not really listening but instead merely waiting. Perhaps my view here is skewed somewhat by my having been a sometime university teacher who has run into many men with what I think of as professor's disease, which gives them a strong propensity not to converse but to lecture — alas, sometimes for a full fifty minutes. (Where else but in teaching, said the Harvard economic historian Alexander Gershenkron, is a man permitted to speak for fifty minutes without being interrupted by his wife?) "One of the most soothing forms of stroking," writes Jessie Bernard, "is simple listening" — at which women, in my experience anyway, seem to do a better job.

Why men more naturally feel a stronger sense of competitiveness than women can perhaps be explained by nurturance. Boys are trained to hold their own and not be bested. Competitive emotions may come quite as naturally to women — the rise of female athletics has shown this — but women are supposed to feel a bit odd at exhibiting them openly, let alone permitting them to get out of hand. When a man meets another man, it is natural for the two to size each other up: Is he smarter than I, more successful, in some way better built to survive the game of life? Tina Fey, the comedian, would disagree; she thinks that girls can bring a sly meanness to their relations with other girls. "Girls," she remarked, "have ways of hurting each other verbally and emotionally that are completely unseen by the naked eye." Women doubtless size up other women, but usually in less direct, more subtle ways: Is her ostensible elegance real, does she offend me in any obvious way, is she someone with a kind heart, might we become friends? Women seem to understand better than men that competition, good for the marketplace, the athletic field, and a few other places, is not so good for friendship.

Women, as Tolstoy noted, can be more selfless and altruistic than men — not always, not inevitably, but in actual practice often enough to make one feel that emotionally they are better equipped for friendship than most men. Might it be their sense of nurturance, which is also called into being by child-bearing and child-rearing, that also makes them understand that friendship requires kindness, careful cultivation, evenhandedness, and generosity of spirit? Again, professional feminists might not like to hear this, but the more that women become like men in their outlook and ambitions, and the more that hedonism and rivalrousness and *amour-propre* play a central role in their consciousness, the more worn become the cables that hold up the bridge of society, and one of the main such cables is, of course, friendship.

# 10

❖

# *Boys Will Be Boys*

IN MEN, WOMEN HAVE a subject of nearly perpetual interest: the foibles, the tastes, the motives, the moods, the peculiar psychology of men are examined by women at various levels of subtlety and at as much length as leisure allows. Men, when they talk about women, are more limited in their range of interest: they either (1) complain about them or (2) exclaim how they wouldn't at all mind bonking them. Broads. Go figure. Next subject.

In Leonard Michaels's novel *The Men's Club,* in which men meet regularly to talk about intimate things, the author has his narrator remark on the good fortune of women in having so much to unite them in friendship. "Anger, identity, politics, rights, wrongs. I envied them. It seemed attractive to be deprived in our society. Deprivation gives you something to fight for, it makes you morally superior."

Friendships among men are decisively different. Most men feel that men and women operate on entirely different psychological systems. Men see themselves as more logical, women as subtler, men as having a surer view of the larger picture, women more neatly concentrated on life's details. Men drive straight ahead, women are more interested in the view out the rearview and side mirrors, not to mention the sunroof. Men, with shorter memories and thicker skins, are more forgiving: all right, so the guy hit on my wife, what the hell, that was five years ago.

Women are longer-suffering and thinner-skinned: imagine her not noticing I lost ten pounds! I have heard it said that often when women are put in positions of (formerly masculine) responsibility, they sometimes turn out to be more rigid, doctrinaire, and unforgiving than men in the same jobs: the problem is that they are doing poor imitations of how they think men in the same position would behave. The more one thinks about these things, the more the differences pile up, and the more it can seem as if men and women are not of different genders but of separate species.

To be friends, men have to get over their natural rivalry with other men. Like stags in a National Geographic film, men like to clash horns, even if no doe is in sight. They like to know, when faced with other men, if they can beat them up, buy and sell them, outwit them, defeat them in some way that, in their minds, is significant if not necessarily decisive.

The primary difference between men and women perhaps has to do with aggression. Men are permitted aggressive behavior, women — even though for a period in the 1980s courses were offered for women in "natural aggression" — are not. Some evolutionary psychologists (among them Lionel Tiger, in his book *Men in Groups*) argue that this harks back to the male role as hunter, the female as child bearer. Whatever the case, a man without some element of aggression tends to be viewed as less than fully a man; a woman with even the slightest element of aggression is automatically viewed as somewhat suspect.

For men to become friends they must somehow prove themselves to each other. What they must prove is their ability to negotiate the rough bumps in life, and they cannot do this without a certain aggressiveness, or at least they must demonstrate the potential for aggression. "Bonding" is a word that had its origins in evolutionary biology and was taken over, then swamped, by pop psychology, but it originally meant, according to Lionel Tiger, "a particular relationship between two or more males such that they react differently to members of their bonding unit as compared to people outside of it." One of the things that bond men together is their equivalent success in the world, which also means the effectiveness of their aggressiveness upon a hostile environment.

Consider a relatively famous recent three-way male friendship, that among literary Englishmen of the same generation: the poet Philip Larkin, the novelist Kingsley Amis, and the historian of Soviet terror Robert Conquest. (Conquest is not so much the odd man out as my brief description of him suggests; he also writes poems, among them some of the most charming blue limericks of the age.) Larkin was the best poet of his time, Amis the most highly regarded English novelist, and Conquest, in *The Great Terror,* the author of one of the most historically significant books of the past century. Larkin and Amis went to university together; Conquest matched both in comic point of view.

Friendships similar to that among these three men are unthinkable among women, and perhaps among American men. Although they were (Conquest is still very much alive) men of considerable intellectual and artistic seriousness, among themselves they remained schoolboys, perhaps no older than age-fifteen schoolboys. They shared an interest in light pornography, spanking and all that (ah, there'll always be an England), as well as a scruffiness and a deliberate loutishness. Larkin could write to Amis about what a waste of time and money it was to court a woman, when it made much more sense and saved five pounds to toss off early in the evening and spend the rest of the night alone, drinking and listening to jazz records. Amis could report to Larkin on his adulteries and his drunkenness. Their anti-female sentiments were unabashed and, if one is not a woman, wickedly funny. Conquest sent them both limericks quite gigglesome in their obscenity. To one another they could mock the pretensions of the famous among their other friends and acquaintances. In short, guy stuff, to a high and amusing if not entirely admirable power, yet of a kind that gave all three of these extraordinary men much pleasure and probably solace.

Difficult, as I say, to picture similar friendships occurring among women. I cannot imagine any intelligent woman being able to sympathize with such characters; nor should she be asked to do so. But men can. It is the giving way to the beast — the highly civilized beast in the Larkin-Amis-Conquest case to be sure, but the beast nonetheless — that most men find amusing if not meritorious. Men are brutes, and the inside joke with Philip Larkin, Kingsley Amis, and Robert Conquest is that even at their exalted level of cultural achievement, brutes they remain.

Not that their brutishness is unattractive to most men, those who want to be, so to say, men among men, among intensely randy and slightly rowdy men. Yet there was at bottom something false about this show of masculine independence among these three Englishmen. Contemptuous of women though Amis, Larkin, and Conquest come off in their letters as being, all three were in thrall to them. Larkin may portray himself as one of nature's true bachelors, yet all his days he seems to have had a steady woman friend and lived in some fear of being trapped by one or the other of them into a full commitment. Conquest has been a many-married man. And Amis, though married only twice, at the end of his life, riddled with crippling phobias (he couldn't fly, he was afraid of the dark), none of them helped by his impressive drinking — Amis came limping back to live with his first wife and her astonishingly tolerant third husband.

Much talk has been expended in recent years about the feminization of modern society. In England and America, many once exclusively male membership clubs have either closed up or — sometimes under political, sometimes under financial, pressure — had to take in women members. Other masculine redoubts — gyms, pubs and saloons, tennis and golf clubs — have also gone the adult equivalent of co-ed. As far back as 1960, C. S. Lewis, a bachelor don at Oxford, complained:

> To the Ancients, Friendship seemed the happiest and most fully of all human loves . . . The modern world ignores it. We admit of course that besides a wife and family a man needs a few "friends." But the very tone of admission, and the sort of acquaintanceships which those who make it would describe as

"friendships," show clearly that what they are talking about has very little to do with that *Philia* which Aristotle classified among the virtues or that *Amicitia* on which Cicero wrote his book. It is something quite marginal; not a main course in life's banquet; a diversion; something that fills up the chinks of one's time.

Brilliant in so many ways as he was, Lewis, though not he alone, missed a central change in modern society: the possibility, never before so widely available, of friendships between men and women, a friendship outside sexual interest. That men and women, husbands and wives, lovers after flames have cooled, can also be dear friends has changed the nature of exclusive male friendship radically. Put briefly, what this has meant is that all time now spent with men is time taken away from women and family (only for lifetime bachelors and homosexual men is this not now true). "Friendship and marriage-and-family are mutually exclusive alternatives," Leon Kass has written in an essay titled "The Beginning of Wisdom." "Friendship (especially male-male bonding) [now] belongs to the way of others."

And yet most men still long for male friendships, if perhaps not such tight, exclusionary friendships as at an earlier time. Certain things men can derive only from other men. One can be unguarded about many things with the woman one loves, but not all. Only with men can one display one's full-frontal vulgarity, to borrow a phrase from the English novelist Frederic Raphael. Only with men can one comfortably say piss, shit, fuck, and corruption (though this, too, seems to be breaking down, and these words, once a masculine preserve, are now, for better and worse, available to women). Only with men can one banter, use raillery, be heavy-handedly ironic, screw off, and be boyishly, stupidly, happily manly.

I recently had lunch with two old friends and a third friend, of less long standing but of similar background — we are all Jewish, all went through Chicago public schools, all are the same age. Much of the lunch, which took place in a Greek restaurant — a "Grecian spoon," as one of us called it — was given over to joking reminiscences of our own and our contemporaries' outrageous behavior as kids and young men — enjoyable, rather standard stuff for us. Only the towel-snapping, you might say, was missing.

In our amiably rambling conversation, one of us mentioned having gone to what looked to be a very expensive wedding. Considering how much it must cost per plate at weddings nowadays, I wondered aloud, how expensive a gift ought one to give? At which point one among us said he knew exactly how much it costs, and then recounted a story about his partially estranged daughter (estranged because his ex-wife long ago poisoned the girl against him) inviting him to her wedding, but not permitting him to sit at the main table with other honored family guests. When he told her this was unacceptable, and said that he wanted nine people from his side of the family also invited, his daughter agreed, but only if he would pay for these nine guests, which he did, at a cost of $1,800.

He apologized for telling this story. It was a tale of injustice — and unarguable injustice, for this man had paid all his daughter's expenses, including those through college, and he is a kind man. And it was of course a sad story, one of family heartbreak. It was also a story outside the otherwise jokey spirit of the lunch. All of us at that table have our problems. But we don't meet to "share" them. Instead we bear them, each on his own; or tell them to our wives or, if we have them, therapists. The lunch picked up again after this incident. When we departed, we left one another laughing as we usually do.

Yet what were we to do about this story except hear its teller out? He would not want us to weep, nor to explain away his daughter's bad behavior. (He had to settle for one of us — me, actually — saying how wretched his daughter's behavior had been.) He may even have regretted telling it, knowing the ruling ethos of general nonseriousness in our group. But tell it he did, and it lay there, like something disagreeable in the punch bowl, until the subject was changed and all was brushed away by laughter.

At another recent lunch, this one with six other men who had pledged the same fraternity as I at the University of Illinois, where I spent my freshman year, I announced the death of one of the twelve members of our pledge class, a gastroenterologist who had been doing academic medicine in San Diego and with whom I had been in touch by e-mail and phone over the past few years. Three fellows at the table said they had not known about his death, which was noted and then, after my remarking on how bravely he seemed to have died, the subject was fairly quickly passed over. The lunch arrangement was a bit unsatisfactory owing to our being seated at a rectangular and not a circular table. I had not seen some of these guys for decades. One of us was a widower. By now three of our pledge brothers had died. Other deaths were recounted; also past surgeries, minor illnesses, aches and pains and memory loss, though these in a joking way. We were all sixty-seven and pleased still to be in the game, on our feet and in action.

Except for one of us reporting that his son-in-law had recently left his daughter and their two children, about which not all that much was said in response, the conservation was mostly about things on the surface of life, about old times, names out of the past, sports, life's passing scene. When, after ninety or so minutes, we left the restaurant, we agreed to meet again in four or five months. Nothing profound had happened; nothing especially interesting had been said. All of us had gotten through life with no more than the usual scars. Yet I had enjoyed myself. I didn't long for deeper talk; the surface of life, the merely superficial, was OK.

Is the talk of men among men superficial by nature or by design? In groups larger than two, it may well be the latter. The novelist Tim Lott has written that for men friendship is a kind of performance art. "You go out and try to entertain each other. You grandstand, you try and get attention, you aim for the largest laugh." For the most part, this happens to match my experience. The question is, why don't I mind it? Might it have something to do with C. S. Lewis's once affirming that his favorite sound in all the world was masculine laughter? Or might it be that men do not all that much crave intimate talk?

One of the things I noted about lunch with my former fraternity brothers is how little these men had gone afield for new friends. Most of them continued to see the friends they had made in high school or college. Some among them had remained close; in fact, two of them had married sisters and become brothers-in-law; two others worked as partners in the same business. They lived in the same few suburbs on Chicago's North Shore. I, who had left the University of Illinois for the University of Chicago, was the only one who had become bookish. Although I retained a few good friends from the old days, most of the male friends I had made since college now had interests similar to mine, lived in other cities and countries, were often ten or so years older or much younger than I.

I have at present only one female friend with whom I can talk easily about intellectual things in a free-swinging way: culture, politics at the level of the ideological, literary questions. She is a hardy character, whose intellectual specialty is pointing out how others have overlooked the obvious: "Women are sexual objects, hell," she said to me early in the rise of feminism. "I never slept with anyone I didn't want to sleep with." A certain toughness is required for serious intellectual talk, which can be combative. Not everyone has a hide hard enough to be told that they are obtuse, without penetration, flat-out wrong about things they take seriously. With no basis for evidence other than my instinct, my sense is that men can take this kind of combative talk more easily than most women.

Intellectuality is to me what golf or art collecting is to someone else: a central interest that serves as an organizing principle of my life. I have long been naturally attracted to bookish people, though not exclusively; some among them are similarly attracted to me. But if something resembling a friendship is to develop between us, an element beyond mere intellectual interest has to enter in. This usually includes my sense of the other person's courage in holding unfashionable beliefs, his perceptiveness, his depth, his integrity. But these, I recognize, are public qualities.

If some of my best friends are intellectuals, their intellectuality alone is not what I chiefly prize in them. What I prize are the qualities above intellect—kindness, generosity, amused self-deprecation. I have a friendship with a man who, because he lives in Maine and I in Chicago, I see perhaps once, maybe twice a year. We have known each other for more than forty years. Whenever we meet alone I am reminded of why I like him so. Our friendship, if I may put it thus, is beyond intimacy. We don't really need it. We each know what the other has and has not accomplished in life; we know who are the con men and who the heroic figures in our line of work; we have a similar sense of what is hilarious in the world (other people's pretensions to virtue being high among items in this category); we know the clock is running (he is nine years older than I) and that our ages have begun to make us less central, more peripheral characters — all these things we know in common. When we are alone talking, I do not have to worry about definitions of friendship; I am living in it. When last we met, for a Chinese dinner, I told him how I wished we could meet for dinner at least once a week. I don't believe we should ever run out of things to talk about or run out of good feelings for each other.

I have another friend whom I met when we were both in our early fifties. Although we grew up in different cities in the Midwest, our backgrounds — Jewish, lower-middle-class, big-city wiseguy — are similar. He taught philosophy for a while, then went into business; now retired, he retains an interest in intellectual things and reads widely, especially novels. Our politics are not the same. Neither are our temperaments. He is a man who needs no schedule; he was able to kick back and chill out long before either of these phrases was invented. If he is reading a good book, he might stay up until three A.M. to finish it, and sleep until noon the next day. If I, who go to bed most nights at ten, do not easily fall asleep, I start to worry about the following day being shot.

Our style with each other is teasing, aggressive, jokey, ironic. He might remark on a beautiful woman, and I will ask why she would ever be interested in a man of advancing middle age, with all the accompanying symptoms of deterioration, such as he shows. We make two-dollar bets on tennis, basketball, and football games, bets I dislike losing because he gloats so when he wins. We speak seriously only when we talk about children, specifically his son of fifteen (born late in his life) and my granddaughter of sixteen. Separated in an amicable divorce from his wife, he is an earnest and extremely good father; having a son to worry about gives his often frivolous-seeming personality a useful moral ballast.

In our friendship we make few demands of each other. We have never loaned each other money, asked anything of each other in the way of a real sacrifice. Usually we get together once a week for lunch or dinner. Our mutual understanding, with the overlays of irony in our conversations, is near perfect. Within this shared irony, our intimacy grows and flourishes without need of deeper roots. For the most part, we agree in our judgments of people we know. We are each capable of saying things causing the other to laugh very hard. When he told me that an acquaintance of ours, a man of cold personality, had a detached retina, I asked him how the doctors could be sure that his retina wasn't firmly in place and everything else about him was detached.

We seldom talk about ourselves in an earnest manner. He knows a vast deal more about philosophy and religion, particularly about the religion we were both born into, than I. I happened to tell him that, though I was agnostic on the subject of God, I tried to live my life as if God existed and figured to reward or punish me at the end of my game. "Ah," he said, "Pascal's wager." "Yes," I replied, "but Pascal never tells us that the odds on God's existence are five-to-two against." To which he responded, "And you, no doubt, also want points."

We play each other like old cellos. Each of us knows, socially, all the other's moves. We share an unspoken understanding that, in good measure, life is a silly play in which we have insignificant parts, growing more insignificant the older we grow. I enjoy the sight of him. I'm never disappointed when it is he who calls me on the phone. I hope he feels something of the same when he picks up the phone and I am on the other end. I hope he feels of me, as I do of him, quietly but pleasingly charmed at the notion that we are friends.

. . .

Despite some of the experiences I have just described — and I could add a number of others — ours is not thought to be an especially good age for male friendships. As mentioned earlier, women have been able to find common ground for friendship around the unjust deprivations of the past. They have had obvious reasons for uniting against old-line job and other forms of discrimination, obvious and subtle. They have also been integrated into what were once exclusively masculine domains: men's clubs, athletic clubs, executive boardrooms, law firms, and many other places. At one point there was even talk of making pool, once the domain of working-class men and the lumpenproletariat, a family game. For a time, cigar clubs opened in New York and elsewhere as a new exclusively male domain, but at the moment they don't look to have much staying power. The greater emphasis on the central importance of family over friendly life has cut into the informal institution of boys' night out, for poker, bowling, the lodge meeting, softball.

Something on the order of a men's movement was under way ten or fifteen years ago. The poet Robert Bly's *Iron John* was published in 1990; the book is a rather vague and gaseous attempt to help men find the old confident masculinity taken from them by upbringings that, Bly contends, left them depressed or empty. "The journey most American men have taken into softness, or receptivity, or 'development of the feminine side,' has been an immensely valuable journey," Bly wrote, "but more travel lies ahead." The road Bly sets out in his book is strewn with a mélange of myths, legends, and hope of finding the inner warrior, thought to be part of the natural heritage of every man. It's empty stuff, near as I can make out, but then what should one expect of a book that instructs one on how to be manly?

The men's movement was formed not so much in opposition to the women's movement, but because men were thought to be psychologically rudderless. The women's movement supposedly helped demonstrate this to them. One doesn't hear much about the men's movement nowadays, perhaps because every movement has to have a direction, and it was never very clear — as it was clearer with the women's movement — in what direction it ought to be headed. For Bly, the direction was toward a return to an old-fashioned—actually medieval—manhood, with sensitivity to women added. As the song had it, "Nice work if you can get it." But it remains far from clear if you really can get it, no matter how hard you try. And if you have to try, it probably isn't worth it anyhow.

That homosexual men can teach poor heterosexual men a thing or two is another item that has come to the fore of late. The journalist Andrew Sullivan, in *Love Undetected*, claims that gay men have "been able to sustain a society of friendship that is, for the most part, unequaled by almost any other part of society. Heterosexual women have long sustained it, of course, when their familial responsibilities have not overwhelmed them. But heterosexual men, to their great spiritual and emotional impoverishment, have for far too long let it pass them by."

Sullivan feels that the model of homosexual friendship could well provide a way for heterosexual men to find a return to "the possibilities of intimacy and support that friendship offers, to expand the range of relationships and connections that every heterosexual person can achieve." But do most men long for the kinds of intimacies and support that Sullivan finds so rewarding in the gay world? My sense is that, in a therapeutic age, such things are made to seem the road to true happiness: I tell you my darkest secrets and terrors, and you tell me that you are there for me and always will be. Hug, and dissolve to credits.

Why do I find this not only unhelpful but unappealing? Am I one of those men Sullivan refers to whose emotional life has been clogged by "the etiolated and awkward [masculine] gestures of the 1950s"? Perhaps so, but such gestures remain for me inextricably tied to my core conception of adulthood, manliness, and the acceptance of a tragic view of life. In the line of intimacy, I have no wish to be like women, or gay men, or successful therapy patients. I am simply and utterly unable to find any attraction to the intimacy, outside my own family life, that such a path to my putatively deeper self promises, and I hope this sentence won't cause my friends to stage an intervention for me.

I wonder, too, if the recent phenomenon of men everywhere

hugging one another has grown out of this putative masculine need for greater intimacy. Men hugging each other, in greeting or departing, began, I believe, in show biz. Sammy Davis, Jr., was a great hugger; people of a certain age will recall the photographs of his hugging Richard Nixon, one of the least huggable of men in all of Western civilization. Jesse Jackson, probably to his political regret, hugged Yasir Arafat. Athletes soon took it up: the post-touchdown hug became standard jock congratulatory procedure. Now all the boys are doing it. In *David Copperfield*, young David, as punishment for getting into a fight, is made to wear a sign at school that reads "He bites." I shouldn't myself mind wearing a small sign that reads "Doesn't hug. Will accept hearty handshakes."

Meanwhile, every man has those moods when he longs for purely masculine company. Samuel Johnson, though a married man until his fifties, when his twenty-years-older-than-he wife died, used to speak of going out for "a frisk" with his largish circle of male friends. "I have a mind to frisk with you gentlemen this evening," he would say. A Johnsonian frisk might include a session at one of his male clubs, a pub crawl, a late dinner, all including bouts of conversational jousting, at which he was supreme.

Men seem to need a frisk, of various kinds, more than do women. They also have tastes that women cannot be expected or asked to share. Often these tastes are for the coarse. I never met a woman who finds the comedian Rodney Dangerfield even faintly amusing; most women can live nicely without the writing of H. L. Mencken and the movies of W. C. Fields; and Hemingway tends not to light too many female fires. In Norman Rush's novel *Mating*, the female narrator remarks: "One thing you distinctly never want to hear a man you're interested in say softly is that his favorite book in the whole world is [Doris Lessing's] *The Golden Notebook*. Here you are dealing with a liar from the black lagoon and it's time to start feeling in your purse for car fare." Men's and women's tastes differ, not down the line, not always, but often and clearly enough to make life much more interesting than otherwise.

• • •

In this chapter I seem to have made men out to be amusing (though not highly) louts if not savages, while in the preceding chapter I've made women out to be little saints of sensitivity. Neither is of course strictly true. All I wish to emphasize is that the two operate under different modes, styles, and codes of friendship. Despite the spirit of the day, most men do not wish to be hugged by other men. Nor do they wish to turn their friendships into unpaid therapy sessions. Except on their deathbeds, men generally cannot tell other men how much they like them, or how much their friendship means to them. A man can do so, but at the risk of reducing the quality of the friendship. Reticence is of the essence in masculine friendship, long has been, and probably ought to continue to be.

What I think most men look for in their male friendships is an outlet of sorts in which they can slip the responsible roles they play elsewhere — as workers, husbands, fathers — and conform only to their uncomplicated pleasures and whims. They don't, for example, really want to talk about sex but only to fantasize briefly about it. In a masculine friendship earnestness is all very well, but it needs regular refreshment by wit and whimsy and sometimes simple crudity. In their friendships, most men prefer to keep things fairly superficial, with only occasional dives into the depths.

Strong disagreement about politics, about religious belief, and about justice in life is possible in masculine friendships — perhaps wider disagreement is possible here, as I've suggested, than in feminine friendships — but agreement on core matters is of course what makes friendships worth maintaining. At this core are such questions as how seriously to take the world, how far a man's responsibility should extend, and how well one holds up under the fire of the inevitable blows dealt out by life.

On the subject of these blows, Stuart Miller, the author of *Men and Friendship,* asked men four of what he terms "impossible questions" to test the depth of their male friendships:

1. If your friend called you at two in the morning and said, "I'm out here by the highway and I need you to come

at once and help me bury a body, no questions asked," would you go?

2. If your friend needed to move in with you for a year, would you receive him?

3. If your friend asked you to mortgage your home for him, would you do it?

4. If your friend went crazy, difficult-crazy, would you keep him out of the hands of mental health authorities by taking care of him for as long as it took?

I'm not sure what it says about me, but for five or six of my closest friends I would answer yes to the first question and an unhesitating no to everyone on the other three questions. Perhaps it says that I am capable of brief acts of stupid generosity and intense loyalty, with an added willingness to commit a crime, but am not to be counted on for the long pull required by serious friendship. Sorry.

*Men and Friendship* is also about the quest of its author, a married man, for deep — perhaps intense is the more precise word — masculine friendship. Stuart Miller is a man with a Ph.D. from Yale, a novelist, and someone who has held important-sounding jobs; he is a man of reasonably wide culture and upper-middle-class tastes. "Men have been taught to run in shrieking fear from tenderness," he writes. "I tell myself that we will need real strength to bring it back." In his closing pages he offers a list of some of the requirements for masculine friendship, among them "being willing to acknowledge the hurt of your own loneliness"; "being willing to be hurt, repeatedly, by people you befriend"; "acting forthrightly with your friend and with the courage of your own delicate needs and desires by living the openness, generosity, and commitment you want from him."

"Hey, Stuart," I want to say to him, imagining his calling me on the phone after I have just read this, "the next couple of months or so are kind of crowded for me. I'll get back to you." Click.

I wonder if many men, longing intensely for masculine

friendship in the manner of Stuart Miller, haven't idealized their youth, recalling it filled with seamless, passionate friendships. Some of these friendships — twin Huck Finns on a raft, riding on a river of adult obtuseness — may have come close actually to having existed. My own boyhood memories of friendship are joyous: filled with laughter and goofy adventure and a sense of complicity against the world. Grand as these friendships were, part of the pleasure in them was owing to the near complete irresponsibility of life in all its other departments. One could in those days give everything to friendship, and friendship was itself everything — it was pretty much what life was about. And damn fine it was for those to whom friendship came easily — and heartbreaking for those to whom it didn't come at all.

But perfect friendships of the kind one remembers — imagines? — having had in youth are, given the nature of adult life, no longer attainable. Too many other demands are made on adult men to give friendship the same attention it received when young; flaws that were more easily overlooked when one was a kid grow larger and more emphatic with the onset of years. As an adolescent, I was a middle-distance friend of a slightly older boy who was a sexual braggart; when I encountered him again when we were both in our sixties, and he was still bragging about his sexual conquests, I found such talk irritating and chose not to see him again.

The frisking Samuel Johnson was a man for whom friendship meant a great deal. He was also a man who, so to say, put his money where his sentiments were. He was kind and generous to the many people he met and befriended on his many frisks, and these included several people, men and women, well below him socially and intellectually, including a few with major disabilities. Some of these people Johnson regarded as "companions," others as "intimate friends." To be an intimate friend of Johnson's required rough intellectual parity, the achievement of which, given the capacious grandeur of Johnson's mind, could not have been easy.

In friendship, Samuel Johnson was very much an Aristotelian. Like Aristotle, he felt the highest form of friendship was between equals, not least equals in the realm of virtue.

Johnson allowed that we are sometimes "induced to love those we cannot esteem" and "compelled to esteem those we cannot love." But in true Aristotelian/Johnsonian friendship, love and esteem must both be present, virtue binding the two together. "When Virtue kindred Virtue meet," he wrote in his poem of 1743, "Friendship: An Ode," "And sister souls together join."

Johnson was no easier to compete with in the realm of virtue than he was in that of intellect. He gave away his last pennies to beggars, brought ill strangers he found in the streets home to live with him. He would probably have answered the last three of Stuart Miller's "impossible questions" positively, without the least hesitation, and answered the first negatively — the reverse of my showing. Taking his Christianity with the utmost seriousness, Samuel Johnson, had he been a Catholic, would long ago have been made, and deservedly so, a saint.

If friendship in the high Aristotelian sense entails equality of intellect and virtue, wasn't Samuel Johnson flat out of luck, being unable to find anyone anywhere near as good as he? He, it turns out, didn't feel so, and his various comments and letters suggest that he found such a friend in a man twenty years younger than he, Edmund Burke, the great political writer and orator.

Their minds were of a very different order: Johnson's was profound; Burke's, though by no means shallow, ran more to brilliance. Both were dazzling talkers, and on an occasion when Johnson was ill, he remarked that he couldn't possibly entertain Burke because he needed to be in top fettle to carry on a conversation with him. He also allowed that, since they were both regarded as conversational performers, when together they sometimes overstated themselves because they became swept away by the pleasures of verbal combat.

Burke, like Johnson, was exceedingly generous; he was also, from all reports, again like Johnson, physically fearless. The two men evidently esteemed each other equally. When Burke was peripherally involved in a political scandal, he came in his depression to Johnson, to tell him he was thinking of leaving public life, so that he "should do no ill." To which Johnson replied, "Nor do good either, Sir," and persuaded him to remain. During his final illness, Johnson averred that Burke's company had always been a delight to him. Burke was Johnson's first pall-bearer, and long after his death, when Johnson's name came up in Parliament, Burke said: "Dr. Johnson was a great and good man, his virtues were equal to his transcendent talents, and his friendship I value as the greatest consolation and happiness of my life."

And yet it is unclear how often the two men saw each other. The biographical literature suggests that it wasn't all that frequently, and only rarely did they meet tête-à-tête. Nor could they talk about everything. Johnson was a Tory, Burke a Whig, and politics, important to both men, though perhaps more so to Burke, was ruled out as a subject for discussion when they were together. Johnson could also be critical of Burke's style for being too openly emotional on the floor of Parliament; he also told others that he didn't favor Burke's penchant for punning, which he thought a low form of wit.

I don't wish to devalue what must have been a great friendship between two vastly talented men. I wish only to take a little of the pressure off the ideal of friendship as a seamless, selfless regard of two souls, each for the other. This is not how true friendship works. Even among the best men and the best women — and Samuel Johnson and Edmund Burke were among the very best — friendship, grand though it can be, is always qualified by tact and restraint. Important, I think, never for a moment to forget this.

# 11

❖

## *Petty Details*
## *vs. Eternal Verities*

ODD TO THINK SO, but friendship, like race, had long been under the cruel and wasteful, if unlegislated, rule of segregation. Women had always found friendships with other women, and men with men. But the crossover possibility, that of male-female friendships outside sexual interest, has only in recent years widened and greatly enlarged the realm of friendship in the modern world.

Exceptional people, however, have long enjoyed such friendships. The friendship dearest to Samuel Johnson, for example, was that with neither Edmund Burke nor James Boswell (who was nowhere near his equal), nor that with his wife (whom he loved), but with a woman named Hester Thrale, the wife of Henry Thrale, a successful London brewer. Their friendship began in 1765, when Johnson was fifty-five and Mrs. Thrale twenty-four. The Thrales, in an act of great compassion, rescued Johnson from a deep, possibly suicidal depression and took him to their country home, where he remained for three months, until, his spirits restored, his health regained, he was able to plunge back into life with his former ardor. After this, a room was always kept for Johnson in the Thrales' London and country houses.

By the time she met Johnson, Hester Thrale was an accomplished woman. She spoke French as a child, later acquired Greek and Latin, Italian and Spanish. She wrote poetry, and she and Johnson, early in their friendship, began work on a translation into English of Boethius's *Metres*. She endured twelve pregnancies, from which only four children survived. She was not a beautiful woman; Walter Jackson Bate, Johnson's best biographer, describes her (from portraits) as "very short and birdlike, with a sharp nose, a wide mouth, and large hands . . . But, if not a beauty, she was vivacious, charming, and warm-hearted." She saw to it that Johnson's every physical and psychological need was met. He, in turn, was devoted to her.

What was in this friendship initially for Hester Thrale was perhaps the capture of a lion, for Johnson was already famous as a literary man and his reputation as the greatest talker in England was backed up by repeated performance. What was in it for Samuel Johnson was, at first, a life of an orderly kind that he had never known and within a family that adored him; and, later, a relationship with a person in whom he could confide many of the things that troubled him. Mrs. Thrale's husband was a philanderer, in a way not uncommon to the age and, apparently, not all that troubling to her. Johnson was long a widower. Yet physical love between the two was never considered a possibility.

Hester Thrale catered to Johnson, coddled him, gave him the sense that he had a home. He was playful with her children, respectful of her husband, and provided a seemingly unending flow of charming talk for the family. When, after her husband's death, Hester Thrale allowed love, for an Italian music teacher named Gabriel Mario Piozzi, to trump friendship in her relation with Johnson, it broke his heart: such was the depth of affection he had put into his friendship with her. That friendship was now over, never to be repaired, a shattering blow to the by now elderly Johnson. But a genuinely deep friendship it was, of the kind that sociologists call a "cross-sex friendship," though Samuel Johnson would have smirked, twitched, and then blasted the ugliness of the phrase out of the bloody water.

· · ·

Another famous literary male-female friendship was that in the seventeenth century between Madame de Lafayette (the author of *The Princess of Cleves,* often called the first novel) and the Duc de La Rochefoucauld (the author of the immortal *Maximes*), who lived together — chastely, the presumption has always been — in friendship after her widowhood and his retirement in the twilight of his defeated ambition. Their friend Madame de Sévigné said that "nothing could be compared to the confidence and charm of their friendship." Madame de Sévigné, herself a model of kindness and amiability, had several close friendships with men; La Rochefoucauld, who knew her well, remarked that "she satisfied [my] idea of friendship in all its conditions and qualifications."

Dorothy Parker and Robert Benchley seem to have had a close friendship of nearly perfect equality and without its being soiled by competitiveness on either side, rare in two writers working roughly the same vein of sophisticated comedy. Parker lived more recklessly than Benchley, and he was always around to help pick up the debris from her destructive habits and bad decisions. "Keep this up, Dorothy," he is supposed to have said when visiting her in the hospital after one of her suicide attempts, "and you're going to make yourself very sick."

Closer to our time, Evelyn Waugh, who would have dismissed "cross-sex friendship" as vulgar American sociologese (which of course it is), enjoyed such a friendship with the novelist Nancy Mitford, the author of *Love in a Cold Climate* and other works. They were contemporaries — he was born in 1903, she in 1904 — and she was of the aristocracy, to which he aspired and to which his talent as an artistically and commercially successful novelist eventually gained him entry. Both considered themselves superior, which they doubtless were, but treated each other as equals.

Their friendship began in earnest when Evelyn Waugh's first wife, who was a friend of Nancy Mitford's, left him for another man — a shattering experience — and Mitford showed her allegiance to him. Without many of the ordinary virtues though Waugh was, gratitude appears to have been one he never abandoned. He had friendships with other women — Lady Diana Cooper and Ann Fleming (the wife of Ian Fleming) — but none so rewarding to him (to them both, really) as that with Nancy Mitford.

If she was socially superior to him, he was artistically superior to her. He it was who encouraged her to write, and he who continued to correct her grammar and spelling for the remainder of his life. He did this in letters, and their friendship was largely epistolary, most intensely so between 1939 and 1966, the year of Waugh's death. (Mitford lived on to 1973.) Waugh remarried, when he was thirty-four, to a girl of seventeen; and Mitford married, in her late twenties, an attractive but feckless man named Peter Rodd. Although Waugh and Mitford had their disagreements — his dogmatic Catholicism, the religion to which he had converted, was high on the list of their disputations — they both had a deep appreciation for a style of life, the aristocratic leisure class, that they sensed was well on its way out.

In their letters an intimacy of tone and spirit prevails, sometimes embarrassingly so, as when Nancy Mitford writes to Waugh that "I used to masturbate when I thought about Lady Jane Grey so of course I thought about her constantly and even executed a fine watercolour of her on the scaffold." On display in their friendship was candor given a high-spirited and comic turn. He, for example, could write to her: "My unhealthy affection for my second daughter has waned. I now dislike them all equally. Of children as of procreation — the pleasure momentary, the posture ridiculous, the expense damnable." At one point, he asks her to burn an especially mean letter of his, to which she replies: "What a very rum request. I *especially treasure* your nasty letters, posterity will love them so. However just as you say." Like all good friends, they were lucky in finding each other.

When one considers the Johnson-Thrale and Waugh-Mitford friendships, one realizes that husbands and wives had to show either a good-hearted disinterest or a cold-blooded indifference to allow them to flourish as they did. I bring this up because, as ought to be obvious, marriage is the first potential obstacle to strong male-female friendships. There has to be trust, or (as in the cases of Henry Thrale and Laura Waugh and Peter Rodd) lack of interest in one's marital partner, to permit such friendships to flourish outside the marriage. A jealous husband or wife puts the instant kibosh on the possibility of a deep opposite-sex friendship.

Some might say that there is a prior, less surmountable barrier, hormonal in nature. They would argue that a true relation of any closeness between a man and a woman in which sex isn't, in ways evident or obscure, a prominent factor is simply not possible. In *The Sun Also Rises*, Ernest Hemingway has a character say, "Women made such swell friends. Awfully swell. In the first place, you had to be in love with a woman to have a basis in friendship." Hemingway, often so touchingly poetical a writer, really shouldn't have been permitted to think. In his friendships with women, he seemed to want that common enough male fantasy, a lover with a man's mind and a woman's body. This, though, isn't available.

Hemingway must have thought he came close to this ideal when he began a love affair and then entered into a marriage — his third — with the journalist and novelist Martha Gellhorn. Like almost all relationships based on fantasy, this one, too, was a flop. Gellhorn turned out to be a better man than Hemingway, and didn't choose to go along with the fantasy. "He needed me," she later wrote, "to run his house and to copulate on — I use the word advisedly, not 'with' but 'on.'"

Friendship is different from love. Physical love is about possession; the heat it ignites is nothing like the cool, measured pleasures friendship brings. The two, as I have noted earlier, are best left unmixed. In support of this point, Nietzsche, in *Human, All Too Human*, remarks that "women can form a friendship with a man very well; but to preserve it — to that end a slight physical antipathy will probably help." This much, at least, can be said: once sex, not latent but actual, becomes an element in the relationship, something other than friendship is going on.

An episode of *Seinfeld* deals directly with this question of friends having sex together. Jerry and Elaine, former lovers now friends, are sitting together comfortably one evening in his apartment, discussing the current paucity of sex in each of their lives. The discussion leads them to conclude that their return to enjoying sex with each other need not wreck their satisfying friendship, especially if they are careful not to let things get out of bounds. They lay down a set of rules governing this new relationship, which will keep it on its old nonromantic basis. The aim is to have "that" (sex) while continuing to have "this" (their close but happily casual friendship). "That," it will not surprise anyone to learn, all but kills "this," and at episode's end it is clear that new arrangements will have to be made if their formerly fine friendship is to be reinstated.

Exceptions doubtless exist to this general rule about male-female friendships being unable to survive physical intimacy. A story used to be told about the now forgotten Chicago writer Isaac Rosenfeld, in his day an impressive woman chaser, who was keeping company with a homely woman of wide intellectual interests. A friend asked Rosenfeld, who before then had had many attractive female friends, what was really going on. "Ah," he is reported to have replied, "it's not the sex that interests me, but the conversation afterward, which is dazzling."

The notion that two healthy people of the opposite sex cannot meet regularly and talk about important things without eventually falling into bed with each other is part of the fading but still enduring Freudian heritage. All other Freudian ideas — from the Oedipus complex to feces being symbolic of money — have been laughed out of the court of reason and empirical science, but the notion that at bottom (also at middle and at top) we are sexual beings, ready at the least chance to have at it, has not. A good Freudian is likely to consider most friendships between a man and a woman as erotic, and for that matter close friendships between people of the same sex as homoeroticism, more or less disguised.

A latent libidinal interest in a friend of the other sex doesn't, I think, count. I should be delighted to confirm Freud by reporting that many women, in their need to get me into their beds, have spoiled otherwise deep friendships, but, sad truth to tell, with only one notable exception (thank God) women seem to find me completely resistible. Like most people with any imagination, I have myself speculated on having sex with all sorts of women whom I regard as friends — even speculate on what sex might have been like with now older but still elegant women when they and I were much younger.

But, then, I am a Walter Mitty of the libido. I am also of the school of the *New Yorker* writer Joseph Mitchell, who once, in a strong Carolinian accent, told me: "Joe, I am of a generation that can never consider sex a trivial act. When I was a boy, if you did *ugly* with a girl, her brother might kill you." I always smile when I think of "did *ugly*."

Letty Cottin Pogrebin puts this matter well in her book *Among Friends,* where she writes that "love is always enlarged when two lovers have a friendship, while friendship is usually diminished when two friends become lovers." She also feels that women "must be *desexualized in nonsexual contexts.* We must not be seen as The Female when sex and gender are not relevant." Sex among male and female friends can only, Ms. Pogrebin is too polite to say, fuck everything up.

Another obstacle to male-female friendships is feminism in its intemperate strain, at least as it has developed over the past thirty or so years. Intemperate feminists want to exist on a plane of equality with men — for many maybe rise a bit higher, owing to the virtue they have attained through suffering — while simultaneously doing all they can to undermine the good faith that is necessary to all friendship. Intemperate feminists assume that men bring nothing but low motives to their relations with women: wanting to exploit them in one way or another. The kind of high-intensity, on-the-attack feminism I am talking about here is, I hope, gradually disappearing from the scene, and perhaps still finds a comfortable home only in universities, and its disappearance can only be a boon to male-female friendships, which, like any other kind of friendship, is not possible without a basis in goodwill and trust.

One of the women whom I think of as a dear friend, it occurs to me, may well consider herself close to being a strong feminist

in the sense I have described, though I do not think she quali-
fies. She thinks herself a 1960s girl. Her politics are inevitably
and unabashedly left wing, and her ever voting for even a cen-
trist Republican is unimaginable. She is outspoken to the point
of never holding back, on politics or much else. As for her
nearly inveterate leftism, it must be said that she has earned the
right to it more than most people I know by being easily the
most generous person I've ever met. Her liberality in politics is
matched by the liberality of her spirit: she has worked long
hours for charities, including, every Thanksgiving morning,
serving food at homeless shelters. People in trouble turn to her,
and even when the requests are beyond reason, she does all she
can not to fail them. Part of her generosity is made possible by
her astonishing energy, but a greater part by her ample good
heart.

Propinquity set our friendship in motion: we were neighbors
on the same floor of an apartment building nearly twenty years
ago. She is fourteen years younger than I but feels close to a
contemporary. She prides herself on her hipness, her stylish-
ness, her ability to spot and stay on top of trends, all of which I
find both informative and charming. She frequently brings me
up to speed on the nuttiness of designer culture: informing me,
some years back, for example, that the designer Kate Spade had
licensed someone to manufacture mints with her initials on it.
With her now ex-husband, she ran a very successful business.
She's pleased to be able to travel to Europe with only a carry-on
bag for luggage. She craves the action of business, enjoys the
sport of moneymaking.

Our meetings usually include a spell or two of breaking-up
laughter. But also serious talk, lots of it about her son and my
granddaughter, who are friends and less than a year apart in
age, and about the complications of current-day child-rearing.
She now lives in a wealthy suburb, and we talk about how the
very rich live, which in her reading turns out to be, for the most
part, pretty stupidly. We both have an anthropological interest
in status and snobbery. We are also candid with each other in
money matters. "Honey," she'll say to me, "that jacket — cashmere, no? What'd ya pay for it?" And I'll tell her.

Like a man of strong character, she has never suggested, let alone admitted, any sense of fear in confronting the world, which, since her divorce, she has done quite on her own. She is high-spirited and passionate in her approach to life, and I admire her courage. She is not someone to be pushed around; she takes the absolute minimum of crap (we all, alas, are called upon to take some); she is a presence in any room in which she stands. Beyond this, she sees life as an adventure, in the way many men, by the time they get to thirty, no longer do. She is always on the attack.

Glad as I am that she is my friend, pleasing though it might have been when I was much younger to have been her lover, I cannot imagine being married to her. Her energy would have driven me into the ground. I also think that she is someone who doesn't require a critical or reflective man, both of which I fancy myself to be. Much as we like each other, I suspect she feels much the same: we are best as good friends.

I must be attracted to women with courage, for another close female friend of mine also seems notable for this quality. She and I go back to grammar school together, though our lives took separate turns after high school. We also have membership in the same sad fraternity of those who have buried children, the older of her sons having been killed, in his twenties, in a car crash. We are also fellow graduates of the institution of divorce, each having survived a bad first marriage, hers under circumstances much rougher than mine. She worked at a secretarial job for years while bringing up her two sons — a delinquent (in all senses of the word) ex-husband did little to help. I, too, brought up two sons on my own. We don't want for things in common.

She was prevented from going to college by a father who, in the bad old days, thought his daughters did not require any education beyond high school, having bred them for marriage. She is a reader of good novels and other books. She does not seem underconfident for not having been allowed to go to college, only slightly cheated out of something she would have enjoyed and at which she would probably have been quite good. She has strong views and is always on the qui vive for snobbery.

She also loves to mock the comic materialism of many of the girls we went to high school with who are now into high-line Armani and heavy-duty cosmetic surgery. She and I were both popular kids in the social beehive of our large high school. I remember boys being crazy about her.

She is small and dresses with care. I have succeeded in gently kidding her out of making quotation marks in speech with her fingers. ("This neighborhood, you will recall," I tell her, "is zoned No Fingerquotes.") We find nothing about which to argue. We meet about every two months, in the late mornings, for coffee or tea, usually for two hours. (We meet once a year as a foursome, with her husband and my wife.) We seem never to run out of things to talk about: grandchildren, the destinies of our old classmates, the condition of our no-longer-dazzling bodies. I'm not sure much of shattering interest gets said by either of us, yet I always come away from my meetings with her feeling pleased, a bit happier with the world. It may derive from her company giving me a sense of the continuity between my long-ago past and today. There is, finally, a quality to the friendship that I could never hope to find with a man.

Another dear woman friend of mine is, alas, long gone. Ours began as a professional relationship. She was perhaps two or three years older than I. We met about twenty-five times before her death, at sixty. We spoke many more times than that over the telephone. She was witty. She was not pretty, did not have good skin, fine hair, elegant features. She smoked heavily. Much of the time she seemed beyond normal vanity. Once I was in her office and she got up and her blouse, a few buttons undone, was not tucked into her skirt. "Tuck that shirt in, kid," I remarked, "I'm sending you in for the second half." I could say things like that to her. I imagined her living in an apartment in great disarray.

All she had was a beautiful mind. She was amusing in an original way. She said remarkable things, which people remember and often quote. Once, attending a meeting of old members of the American Communist Party, she said to her companion, "Do you realize that everyone in this room is the cause of heartbreak in his family?" Complaining of the vast number of typographical errors in the world, she said, "You'd think they would catch them on the 'gallows.'" She was wonderful with language: knew Yiddish; used French artfully; would haul up lovely English words like "estaminet," which she used to great comic effect.

As a young woman, she published a small number of brilliant articles, and then — bang! — the gate came down and she began to suffer a writer's block from which she never recovered. If not being able to do again what one once did so splendidly wasn't suffering enough, she'd made a bad marriage to a writer, a perfect bigot of virtue, who after their divorce and again after her death wrote cruelly about her. But (I can hear her saying this phrase in an immigrant's Jewish accent) "it shouldn't be a total loss": the marriage produced a daughter whom she raised alone and loved beyond all else in the world. Still, hers cannot have been an easy life.

I would often come to New York, where she lived and worked, and not call on her; months would go by when we did not speak. But whenever we were together or spoke over the phone, I felt immediately at ease, at home, with a friend. If I found myself at a cultural event and she was there, I would gravitate to her, seeking safe harbor. Her wit could be devastating in private, but in public she was hesitant, a touch shy. I have no notion whether she liked me anywhere near as much as I liked her.

I don't recall our ever talking about anything deep. A lot of our conversation was comic. She would sometimes leave wild harangues, done in various foreign accents, on my voice mail, addressing me by my last name and threatening me in a menacing way for not being at my desk and working, as any decent human being ought to be at this time of day.

When she died, I felt a loss that has lingered longer than that of many people I've known whom I thought I was much closer to than I was to her. Why? I ask myself. Hers was a strong personality, of course; it left an impress. But more than that, I felt in her a kinship. I felt with her, as Valéry says he felt with very few people, "the sense of being at complete liberty . . . limited only by a fine feeling of proper restraint." We shared something un-spoken, but what?

C. S. Lewis, in *The Four Loves,* remarks that "friends see the same truth," or at least "care about the same truth." What was our truth? We were both intellectuals, working among intellectuals, but we were also something more and less than intellectuals. We couldn't take the notion of ideas altogether seriously. Neither of us ever spoke about it, but we both sensed that, while there were ideas worth fighting for — and that admirable men and women had died for certain worthy ideas — there was also something higher than ideas: we understood that life's real truths were to be found in feelings, instincts, the heart, and not in ideas or in anything else that ends in "ism."

The closest she ever came to confessing to me was to report that her daughter knew that the quickest way to drive her bonkers was to say, when they argued about some domestic matter, "I sense rage, Mother." Our friendship relied on candor instead of confession. She was not someone I would have dreamed of speaking falsely to, for she would, I'm certain, have cut me down on the spot, or else mocked my falsity to others. A savvy friend can sometimes serve as a fine censor without having to say a word.

Two other women whom I consider friends were former students of mine. Now in their forties, both are married and devoted to being mothers. When young, one could pass for a Sally Fields impersonator, the other a dark, Rebecca-at-the-well Jewish beauty. As they sat in my classrooms, both displayed high intelligence, seriousness, and a restrained but obvious distaste for intellectual nonsense.

One of them told me one day at lunch that she had become engaged. "I never thought I'd marry a nice man," she said, in a statement I thought startling but did not ask to have explained. I had not met her future husband, but when I went to her wedding, as the processional began, I looked back and saw that her soon-to-be husband, a handsome man, dragged his legs as he walked down the aisle, the result of cerebral palsy. My heart leapt, I nearly wept, as I thought how much I loved this girl for having the courage and clarity to look beyond the merely physical, to love a man for his kindness and generosity of spirit and not let other things stand in the way.

One of these women lives in Cincinnati, one in Los Angeles. I see them too infrequently. But when I am with them again, after even long absences, it is as if we've not been apart. Quickly crashing the gates of formality, I find myself speaking openly with each of them, as if we were contemporaries and go way back together, which by now we do. They are women of wit and appreciation for wit — people who do not miss much. One works in journalism, the other writes occasional literary criticism. I still feel mildly protective of both — a throwback, I suppose, to my once having been their teacher. I'm not sure what this says about my friendship with either, but I wish each had been my daughter-in-law. This is a complicated statement, considering that I have only one son, to whom, foolish fellow that I am, I neglected to introduce either of them.

I hope these brief portraits of some of the women whom I consider friends do not come off as too Hallmarkian or as bits from *Esquire* magazine's "Women We Love" issue. The fact is that a man can say "I adore her" about a woman more appropriately than one can say the same about a man, and often the emotions one feels about smart, charming, courageous women are close to adoration.

In *Among Friends,* Letty Cottin Pogrebin notes that "the more women friends a man has, the higher his self-esteem." Self-esteem has not been my goal in life, but I am pleased to think that such women as I've described above — and I hope a few others — count me among their friends.

As a younger man, I had a few close friendships with young women, but none felt quite so free and easy as those I have today, in late middle age. I do not concede the Freudians any ground when I say that a man can best enjoy close, nonromantic friendships with women after he has reached a certain age, which is a fact that ought to be put on the credit side of the account book one keeps on the benefits and detractions of aging.

And yet one wonders if the ability of even the young to have nonromantic friendships with people of the opposite sex isn't also changing. In his story "The Briefcase," Isaac Bashevis Singer, one of the most sex-minded writers of the last century, apropos of the complications of his main character's love life, notes: "How right the younger generation was — they no longer demanded faithfulness and they were putting an end to jealousy. Ninety-nine and nine-tenths of our so-called instincts are inculcated by social hypnosis."

But the world has gone beyond Singer's imagination in throwing the young together in ways he could not predict. One wonders, given the new arrangements of the young of both sexes in sharing dormitories, including bathrooms, during college years and later sharing apartments in which nothing sexual is going on, if we haven't already arrived at a minuscule change in human nature. As a scruffy old sex dog, I have my doubts; human nature is not as easily changed as all that. Yet lots of young heterosexual men and women do share apartments, usually for financial reasons, without things going in the direction I, as a young man in a less free time, would devoutly have liked them to have gone.

Most men and women now beyond sixty have probably known opposite-sex friendships only in the context of meeting with other married couples. True couples friendships, involving all four persons equally, are not easily brought off, for, as I noted earlier, in them not merely two but four people must like one another with a reasonably high degree of reciprocity of good feeling all around. I have friends whom I see without their wives because this reciprocity doesn't extend to all four of us. I also know some couples where I find the wife much more interesting than the husband. With such couples, for me the most discouraging moment of any evening is when, as seems frequently to happen, the conversation divides, with men talking to men, and women to women, exclusively. I dislike that moment a lot, and always do what I can, by way of small social engineering involving seating, to prevent its happening.

In his memoir *A Tale of Love and Darkness*, the Israeli writer Amos Oz speaks about his widowed grandfather's great charm for women. The reason behind this charm turns out to have been that, when he was with a woman, "He listened. He did not just politely pretend to listen, while impatiently waiting for her to finish what she was saying and shut up . . . He did not pretend to be interested or entertained . . . He was in no hurry, and he never rushed her. He would wait for her to finish . . . There are many men around who love sex but hate women . . . My grandfather, I believe, loved both."

In the Elizabeth Gaskell novel *Wives and Daughters,* the character Lady Cumnor remarks, "You men concern yourselves with the eternal verities; we women are content to ponder the petty things in life." The petty things in life include merely the careful observation of details, the nuances of human personality and character, the chemistry and dynamics of human relationships. As for those eternal verities, we all know how far we men have come in understanding them. Lady Cumnor, in saying what she did, couldn't, of course, have been more ironic.

# 12

❖

## *Disparate Friends*

ONE OF THE CHIEF REASONS that women were left out of classical accounts of friendship is that equality was everywhere assumed to be a major component of friendship — and in this regard women, politically and in all the ways that followed from the absence of political equality, simply didn't qualify. But there are other kinds of inequality, not to speak of the striking differences in the cards dealt by life, that present rocky shoals for friendship to navigate.

In most accounts of friendship, equality, as we have seen, is indeed everywhere assumed to be central: the starting point, the continuing condition, the sine qua non for maintaining friendship. Aristotle writes that perfect friendship is the "friendship of men who are good and alike in excellence"; he also writes that "friendship is said to be equality." Others have said that friends need not be of equal station in life, but that within the friendship equality must reign — by which is meant that, within the closed realm of friendship, any advantages of power or prestige enjoyed by one or the other of two friends has to be suspended. "Friendships," as Graham A. Allan has written, "are relationships of equality in that friends are accepted as being equal within the relationship. There is no hierarchy in friendship, no differentiation." As usual in matters to do with friendship, the answer is true *and* false, yes *and* no, and above all *maybe*.

One might think that the very nature of friendship not only

implies but also assumes equality. Friendship, in essence, confers equality on the person chosen as friend; part of the honor of being selected as the friend of someone powerful, famous, or otherwise notable is that it allows one to assume that this person considers you his peer. It is in this sense, I suppose, that people think of friendship as self-affirming. If this or that important person wants me as a friend, then, *begorra,* I must be a pretty grand fellow in my own right. But not necessarily so; not even usually so.

Going in quite the reverse direction, when Francis Bacon wrote that "there is little friendship in the world, and least of all between equals," his point was that equality can also breed rivalry. For this reason, it is not uncommon to discover that the two best novelists, painters, composers, or critics working at any one time dislike each other intensely. Equality, then, far from being necessary to friendship, can also in some cases be an obstacle to it.

Many friendships exist in which inequality is, if unspoken, nevertheless assumed. There are what I think of as hold-my-coat friendships. In such friendships, one person is presumed dominant; Achilles over Patroclus, Don Quixote over Sancho Panza (though the latter is the smarter, more sensible fellow), Wonder Woman over Etta Candy. Dickens is full of such characters — Herbert Pocket, Tommy Traddles — who are reliable, self-effacing, and devoted, but always the lesser party in their friendships with various Dickensian heroes. If Oscars were given for friendship, all these characters, and many more in real life, would be candidates in the category of Best Supporting Friend.

Perhaps the most famous case of a best supporting friend is that of James Boswell to Samuel Johnson. There was a thirty-one-year difference in the ages of the two men, who met in 1763, when Boswell was twenty-three and Johnson fifty-four. At no point were the two men ever thought equals, least of all by Boswell, who in the closing pages of his biography of Johnson referred to the older man as "Guide, Philosopher, and Friend." What was in the friendship for Boswell was Johnson's sage counsel, the power of his character, and — more exploitatively

—the prospect of writing a book about the only literary critic who may be said to qualify as a genius.

Boswell also knew the limits of the friendship. He was never less than deferential in the presence of the older man. To his friend William Temple, Boswell wrote of Johnson: "Between ourselves, he is not apt to encourage one to *share* reputation with himself." Johnson also reserved the right to tell Boswell off when his friendship became oppressive: "You have but two topics, yourself and me," he once told him, "and I'm sick of both." Yet the friendship was real, with each man deriving pleasure and comfort from it, and Boswell the additional reward of a literary fame that would not have been available to him had he not cultivated the friendship of Samuel Johnson in the intense way that ultimately resulted in the great book known as *The Life of Johnson*.

I have played the supporting friend role more than once in life. When I did so, it was usually when I was the younger person in a friendship. As an adolescent, I was pleased to be in the company of boys a few years older than I, from whom I could learn things about the world. This sometimes entailed my performing services for them not much above the water-boy level. Perhaps I considered it on-the-job training for discovering how the world works, but up to a point I didn't mind, as long as I really was learning things unavailable to me outside their company.

Devotion and selfless loyalty are required of a hold-my-coat or best supporting friend, and I have myself been able to play the role only when something was at stake for me, which immediately eliminates the ideal of Dickensian selfless devotion on my part.

I earlier mentioned a three-year friendship with Saul Bellow in which I played such a role. He was twenty-two years my senior, with much more experience of the world and much greater fame. Most of the time, owing to a charming combination of effrontery and whimsy, he was a lot of fun to be with. He also had things to teach me. Once, when I characterized the behavior of a New York intellectual as exhibiting great "insecurity," he responded by saying, "What's wrong with using a more old-fashioned and precise word like 'cowardice'?" I've long since dropped "insecurity" from my standard vocabulary of motives.

For much of our twenty-year friendship I played a similar role with Edward Shils, whom I met through Saul Bellow. Bellow once reported to me that he and Edward were together when a man who taught with them at the University of Chicago came up to them and chatted for about ten minutes, and when he departed, Edward said to Bellow that he, the man, was obviously suffering from "illusions of equality."

Edward Shils and Saul Bellow were, or at least seemed, for many years the best of friends. Moreover, their friendship seemed in every way appropriate, fit, meet, right. Near contemporaries — Edward was four years older — outside the sciences they were among the two intellectually most impressive men at the University of Chicago, itself during those years perhaps the most intellectually interesting university in North America. One was a (Nobel Prize) novelist with philosophical and social-scientific pretensions, the other a philosophical social scientist (a Balzan Prize winner) who read (and reread) an astonishing number of novels. At the height of their friendship, both were divorced; both specialized in seeing beneath the surface of things; both were wildly funny, often in a deftly, devastatingly cutting way.

By the time I had come on their scene, playing my second violin (dragging my bassoon may be more like it), the Bellow-Shils friendship was beginning to unravel. (More about this in a later chapter.) At the heart of this was Saul Bellow's notion that Edward Shils did not give him the respect he deserved. This was a friendship with a serious equality problem, with Bellow feeling that Shils did not finally consider him an equal.

Before long Saul Bellow broke with me, ostensibly over a politico-literary argument that he created — that is, one that I believe didn't exist — but really because I found myself drawn more and more to Edward Shils, who had become something close to his enemy, bearing out Paul Valéry's remark, quoted earlier, that we can only truly hate someone we once loved.

To show how subtle these matters can get, Edward Shils was a profound admirer of Arnaldo Momigliano, the great historian of the ancient world. When Momigliano became deathly ill, from an exhausted heart, Edward put him up in his apartment, cooked his meals, did his laundry, saw after all his other needs. A friend of Momigliano's, the historian Glen Bowersock, said he had never seen anything quite like this, one great man looking after another; usually it is left to a lesser man to look after a greater in this painstaking fashion. Edward Shils, in this instance, never shied away from the duties of friendship.

My own friendship with Edward was not one of equals, though in my presence he was always gracious enough to pretend it was. The plain fact is that he was smarter, cleverer, much more learned, and wiser than I — and would be right up to his death, at the age of eighty-five, in 1995. His experience of the world was also greater. I didn't mind taking up a supporting role with him because he was generous to me in many ways, because I learned so much from being around him, and because I grew to love him.

But accepting inequality in a friendship is not always easy. One example is the nearly lifelong friendship between the Supreme Court justices Harry A. Blackmun and Warren E. Burger, as revealed not long ago by Justice Blackmun's papers, which were opened to the public early in 2004 and which show a gradual but decisive breakdown of a friendship of many decades, owing, I believe, to perceived inequality on the part of Harry Blackmun.

Growing up, the two men, who had gone to grade school together in Minnesota, were good friends. Through their years of practicing law in Minneapolis, becoming first federal appellate court judges, then Supreme Court justices (Burger was appointed chief justice), this friendship deepened and strengthened. Burger often used Blackmun to test out his ideas and shore up his intellectual doubts, while Blackmun complained to Burger about how tough it was to raise a family on what was then a less than grand judicial salary. Although he preceded him there, Burger was genuinely delighted when Blackmun was appointed to the Supreme Court: "For me it is the beginning of a great career for you — an association which, whatever the decisions, will be a source of constant strength to the Court, the country, and the C.J. [chief justice]" He also wrote, harking back to their boyhood days: "When we had those dreams of 'doing it together' neither of us ever dreamed it would be this way or in this place [the Supreme Court]. It was the practice we wanted."

Thus far, we have only Harry Blackmun's side of this relationship, but clearly something happened to poison his friendship with Warren Burger. "CJ for the first time very cool," Blackmun wrote in 1980, in the diaries he called his chronology. "CJ picks on me in conference," reads an entry for 1985. And when Blackmun returned to his duties after prostate surgery, the small number of majority opinions Chief Justice Burger assigned him to write, he noted, "makes me feel somewhat humiliated not only personally, but publicly." Blackmun's politics shifted somewhat to Burger's left, but something both more trivial and yet deeper than political differences came to divide the men. Little things that Burger did began to irritate him — and sometimes more than irritate him. Blackmun found his old friend frequently going beyond the bounds in his intellectual pretensions, in pushing himself forward for attention, in the way he handled his job generally. Communication between the two men lessened, then became formal, finally tailing off into the remote and distantly intermittent.

Without intending to demean Justice Blackmun, from all accounts a good man, one cannot help but wonder if he wasn't suffering in a slight but insidious way from the feeling of inequality deriving from Burger's being the chief justice, with the additional publicity and glory that brought, over his being merely an associate justice. (Some merely!) Would this have happened if neither man had been appointed chief justice and equality, even in so exalted a place as the Supreme Court, still ruled between them? Did his additional power truly make Warren Burger as obnoxious as his old friend Harry Blackmun sometimes makes him out to be? One cannot know for sure. La Rochefoucauld wrote, "We all have strength enough to withstand the misfortunes of others," but to be able to withstand their successes can, of course, be something else.

I have a friend, of a very sweet and generous nature, born an

orphan, who married a young lawyer who became very successful. The things that money can buy she has: elegant clothes,
luxury cars, a grand house, first-class travel. They become a
problem only when she meets with her old friends from high
school days, friends who have not been so lucky in life's lottery
as she.

When she meets these friends, she told me, she has to dress
with some care — to dress down, in fact. Nor can she mention,
say, having last month been in London for a long weekend. She
avoids talking about new chic restaurants at which she has recently eaten. She likes her old friends, likes them a lot, but feels
she mustn't in any way flaunt her good life before them. Such
inequalities, even in what might otherwise be long-lasting and
solid friendships, can be insidious, she feels, and who is to say
that she is wrong to feel as she does?

Of course no two people are entirely equal, except perhaps
identical twins not yet gone out into the world, where one is
certain in some way to acquire the edge over the other. One person will always have some advantage, however small. Sometimes advantages can be offsetting and balancing: you have
more culture than I, but I have more money than you; or you
are better-looking than I, but I am healthier than you. But most
times they cannot.

Is it possible, for example, for a person of modest means to
be the close friend of a person of great wealth? Perhaps. But it is
easy to see how often money might get in the way. The person
of modest means cannot permit himself to be the guest of his
wealthier friend with any frequency, lest he begin to feel himself
a sponger. The wealthy friend has to be on guard when making
arrangements that include his less well-off friend, lest he ruin
his budget.

A very well-off man told me a few years ago about ordering
four New York Knicks tickets for himself, his wife, and another
couple from a ticket broker for a Tuesday night game against
Portland, and even he was surprised to learn that the cost of the
(quite good) seats was $2,000. I, for one, should not have
wanted to be the husband of the other couple, on the hook for
$1,000 for two tickets to a basketball game. If there was a large

discrepancy in the wealth of two such friends, should the wealthier man, who ordered the tickets, lie about their true price and absorb much of the high cost? Or should he say that he got them for nothing, in return for a favor, so the question of money doesn't come up? Complications set in quickly when disparities in wealth enter into friendships.

A man who travels in richer circles than I told me about a category that he terms "retinue friends," a group clustering around a friend who has made a great financial success, success at the level of owning yachts, private planes, homes in foreign countries. He often invites old friends along on excursions for which he picks up the tab. Whatever the generosity of the man in control of the money, it is plain that in such friendships the man holding the wallet is also the man who makes the plans, sets the schedules, has in every way control of the wheel. Sometimes the auxiliary company can be quite exotic: powerful politicians, show-business folk, famous writers and artists. The others, the retinue, the old friends, go along because of the sheer luxuriousness of the setting. How nice to talk to Lady Thatcher aboard a yacht anchored at Piraeus!

Another friend tells me that a fellow that he went to school with who struck it rich makes it a point every year to take four or five of his male friends from high school days on an all-expenses-paid trip: to Tuscany, to Las Vegas, or elsewhere. He is a good sport about all this, never making any of these old friends feel in the least awkward. And yet, when my friend told me about these trips and about the no-strings-attached generosity of his friend, my own thought was that I would much rather be paying for everyone else than be one of those whose way was paid.

Perhaps more depressing than friendships changed by economic inequality are those having to do with inequality of cultural attainment. This becomes most poignant when it strikes at old friendships. The euphemism to cover this division is "we've grown apart in recent years," when what is really meant is that one friend has developed wider interests, or has become more penetrating about the world, or has become more bookish than the other. When this occurs, all that old friends seem to

have to talk about are former days, which is to say, the paradisia-
cal times when their interests, far from being divergent, were
congruent.

Such discrepancies occur all the more the older the friends
become. Some people, without quite realizing they are doing it,
edge over to the sidelines: they choose not to learn to use com-
puters, see new movies, read recent books. Others are determined to stay in the game. The former are usually to be found
talking about how the time of their youth was superior to the
present. They reject the world, close down the shop. The latter
continue to take the world as a rich, various, often wildly surprising, always amusing place. People with such strongly con-
trasting views, no matter how much personal history they have
in common, no matter how far back together they go, will find
maintaining such a friendship troubling, from either side.

Unequal prestige is another item that can alter a friendship,
or stand in the way of its ever coming to fruition. The world, in
its unending foolishness, will sometimes award a man or
woman prestige for his or her achievements, in various (and
sometimes unworthy) fields. The persons so rewarded are obviously aware of it, and if they are wise they will at all times recall that prestige is a superfluous and often errant thing and that
the world, which awards it, is, as Henry James might have said,
a great ninny. Still, one's own prestige, however pathetic, can be
difficult to set aside. This can be especially troubling when one
is with someone in one's own line of work whom the world has
overlooked.

Greater prestige can be disabling to a friendship, with the
person holding it being rather in the position of the heftier of
two children on a teeter-totter: he can control the game when
he has a mind to do so by the sheer force of his weight. I always
take a prestige count when out in the world, akin to taking a
Kentucky windage reading in rifle marksmanship, because I
think people who feel they have prestige usually have an easily
offended *amour-propre* about it.

Let me quickly confess that I am not always without such a
pathetic sense of self-regard myself. I recall being invited to

lunch by a poet, who obviously wished to befriend me, but who talked through the meal about himself, his small triumphs, his enemies, his good works, his plans for his brilliant future. At the end, I wanted to touch his hand and say, "Forgive me, but you have spoken way too much about yourself, especially in the presence of someone who, in our puny little literary world, is much better known and more important than you. A serious mistake, especially if you plan to have lunch with me again."

The money that often lies behind social class can be a bar to friendship—as witness my friend and her less well-off high school classmates—and sometimes the cultural differences inherent in social class can do the same, even though social class has become less problematic in America than it once was and the well-to-do are far from necessarily more cultured than anyone else. The old WASP culture, for example, is no longer what it used to be, and people who continue to babble about tracing their ancestors to the *Mayflower* are nowadays missing a much bigger boat.

The barriers thrown up against friendship, often appearing in the guise of inequality, can be at least as various as the reasons for friendship itself. The problems of friendship across cultures can be tragic and, when surmounted, heroic. More often than not, though, they go unsurmounted, as underscored in E. M. Forster's *A Passage to India,* where East remains East, West remains West, and the twain scarcely ever meet.

One of the great victims of the racial troubles in America has long been friendship across racial lines. Good to report that things are finally calming down on this front, but for many years friendships between blacks and whites were freighted with lots of extra baggage, and fraught with nervous tensions that could snap things at any moment. In some ways, the burden was on the white party to what one hates to call—so stiffly, so social-scientifically unfriendly is the phrase—interracial friendships.

In more recent years, the inequality, for once, favored, morally, the black friend. In every such friendship, before it could be considered a friendship at all, whites were obliged to prove that they weren't, deep down, or close up, racists. With even the best intentions this isn't always an easy thing. In the attempt to do so, one might well find oneself guarded in one's use of language — "blackmail, black sheep, black mark," I don't think so — and careful about social land mines, which seemed to lie everywhere. The crude fact of race could take the spontaneity out of friendships between blacks and whites as easily as a stock market crash could take the smile out of Christmas.

I myself have had no truly close black friends. I did have a good, middle-distance black friend named Jervis Anderson (he is now dead) a writer born and raised in Jamaica and educated there in schools on the English model. He might have been a closer friend had we both lived in the same city. But Jervis lived in New York, and chose, my sense was, to separate himself even from people he seemed genuinely to like. (Not many people knew, for example, that he had been married.)

Jervis and I would meet when I was in New York. He often wrote for a magazine I edited. He would sometimes call me long distance in Chicago to talk about baseball. He was the only person I know who understood the intricacies of both cricket and baseball. We talked a lot about writers. He was on the staff of *The New Yorker,* and William Shawn, the great editor of that magazine, who was one of Jervis's household gods, was another of his subjects.

Jervis had, early in his career, written a strong and just piece deflating the black racist Eldridge Cleaver, at a time when it took courage for a black writer to do so. But Jervis and I never talked about race. Perhaps, had we been closer friends, we might have discussed it. But I do not regret that we didn't. Not that I think the subject would have been too explosive for two reasonably intelligent men who felt nothing but goodwill toward each other. Instead I preferred to carry on with the assumption that race could be excluded from a good friendship, which is how we conducted ours.

I have another friendship with a black man, who is my age and who went to the same university I did, though he went into the air force before beginning college and we weren't there at the same time. I hope he finds things as comfortable with me as I do with him. Our subjects are sports and the general wackiness of the University of Chicago in our youth. We dress alike, though he more elegantly than I. We laugh a lot in each other's company. We, too, don't go in for bull sessions about race.

One of the best friendships in American literature, that between the boy Huckleberry Finn and Jim, the slave seeking his freedom, of course crosses racial and every other line. All the power in the relationship is in the hands of the boy, who after all could turn Jim in to the authorities at any time. But the beauty of the developing friendship is Huck's gradual but genuine realization of Jim's standing as a human being. The subtle portrayal of this disparate friendship is what gives Mark Twain's novel its claim to greatness. The lesson for students of friendship is that all friendships begin with regard for the next person's dignity, no matter his or her standing in the world.

I have a small number of friends who are gay, and one good friend who is a lesbian. The latter declared herself lesbian in her late forties or early fifties (I cannot recall exactly). She is a person of serious outlook laced with cheerful good humor — and someone who is entirely open about being lesbian. (She is also the mother of two grown sons.) When we speak, which in recent years we have chiefly done over the phone, the fact of her homosexuality does not signify, as the Victorians used to say. Much of our talk is about the goofy shape the world perennially finds itself in, and lots of this results in laughter. She has a strong taste for Jewish jokes.

Of the four gay friends I see, one I have known for decades, another for less than eight years. With the former, the subject of homosexuality — his or that in the world generally — rarely comes up; in fact he has never bothered to say that he is gay. I have always assumed that he assumes that I know this obvious fact about him.

Two of the other men are twenty or so years younger than I. One of them writes about the gay life. The other, perhaps because he is of a younger generation than mine, is not reticent on the matter of sexuality. (He often and easily refers to his partner, though never talks in a detailed way about what used to be known as one's love life.) He sometimes theorizes about it. At a recent meeting, for example, he attributed the reputed promiscuity of gay men to the fact that all men are inherently promiscuous, and in gay relationships, with two men involved, you get a double dose. The point seemed fairly persuasive. I'm pleased that this friend can talk as openly to me about such things as he does — it signals a certain trust in me and a recognition that I am not entirely unworldly, both of which I take as compliments.

Finally, the fourth of these friends has neither mentioned nor suggested he is homosexual. He has chosen not to do so, I believe, because he feels his own sexual proclivities and practices are no one else's damn business, and therefore not up for discussion. Since I happen to believe the same thing of my own sexual proclivities and practices, I admire him all the more for what I take to be his dignified position.

And yet one wonders about candor in this realm. In *Too Brief a Treat*, Truman Capote's published letters, the highly social Capote writes to a wide range of people, from the Hollywood producer David O. Selznick to the wife of the Kansas state police officer who broke the case that was the subject of Capote's best book, *In Cold Blood*. But the frankest and thus the most amusing letters are those Capote wrote to gay friends, who, the letters assume, know things and live their lives in ways radically different from his heterosexual friends, men and women both.

Differences in wealth, upbringing, sexual orientation, race, and ethnicity, all of these matters touch on snobbery. In a less imperfect world, nothing would matter in friendship but a person's intrinsic worth. Yet the world does not figure to become perfect soon, and until it does, everyone must find ways around such differences as the world has set up for men and women as barriers against their becoming friends.

The only way that I know to do so is to practice a subtle and persistent reciprocity. Everyone must try to make of friendship his own utopian country in which no inequalities exist, where the coin of the realm is imaginative sympathy, all competition and rivalrous feelings are strictly outlawed, the oxygen is considerate talk, and the blood circulates best when stimulated by the constant exercise of thoughtfulness, generous impulse, and kindness. The earnest practice of friendship, in short, requires us to be rather better than most of the time we really are.

# 13

❖

## *Cliques and Clans and Communities*

A CLIQUE, according to *Webster's,* is "a narrow, exclusive circle or group of persons," especially one "held together by common interests, views, or purposes." A clan, outside its strict Celtic meaning, is "a group united by common interests or characteristics," and to act clannishly means "tending to associate only with a select group of similar background or status." Pejorative words all, yet most of us, my guess is, have been cliquish and clannish for the better part of our lives, finding our friends and much of our social life comfortably within cliques and clans.

I am American, midwestern, middle class (34 percent income bracket), middle-aged (latish), middling educated (a bachelor's degree), and Jewish. I also have a fairly wide-ranging interest in culture, in literature and music more than in visual arts, but also in sports and movies. These components of what might be called my sociological profile have determined, to a large extent, the kinds of friends I have had and still do have. But of all the items mentioned above, I wonder if my being Jewish hasn't most affected my choice of friends. I do not seek out other Jews as friends, but Jewish nonetheless a preponderant number of my friends have been and remain. I, it turns out, may be more clannish than cliquish.

I am not, let me quickly insert, religious in any formal way. I belong to no synagogue or church, and have never thought of converting or becoming more serious about the religion into which I was born. I think about God a good deal, but I have only to enter a synagogue (or a church), and God is gone from my mind. My status as a Jew has a minimal amount to do with Judaism and everything to do with Jewishness, or ethnic content. I have been married to two non-Jewish women, neither of whom, given my own religious slackness, did it ever occur to me to ask to convert to the religion of my birth.

Some people do not include ethnicity in their estimates of people, but I am not among them. Ethnicity permeates my social thinking. He's very lively for a Swede, I find myself thinking upon meeting a man named Joe Swanson. "What do you expect, she's a Hungarian," I said when a friend reported a late-life marriage that went belly-up after four months. I've also said, or thought: For a German, he's fairly witty. Even for a midwestern wasp, he's boring.

There are no ethnic groups that fall outside the wide compass of my friendship; I actually have two good friends, a man and a woman, not married to each other, who are Romanians. (The old joke about the difference between a Hungarian and a Romanian is that each will sell you his grandmother, but the Romanian won't deliver.) I think it imperceptive, even in the name of great tolerance, not to consider ethnic background as part of one's appraisal of a person who is a potential friend. Surely it cannot be without meaning that one grew up in America in a Greek or Italian or Lithuanian or Korean or Chinese or Japanese household.

In *The Sexual Organization of the City,* Edward O. Laumann and his coeditors assert that the search for sexual partners among singles tends to be made in large part through ethnic and social class channels, with sexual encounters outside these channels much more the exception than the rule. One might think that in sexual matters, the exoticism of the Other might be an enticement. But apparently not, at least statistically. Cliché though it indubitably is, people seem to feel overwhelmingly more comfortable among their own kind.

I have Jewish friends for whom the next person's being Jewish or not is of no moment, or so they tell me. A person's being Jewish is for me not by any stretch a sine qua non for friendship, but as I say, the bald fact remains that a large number of my friends do happen to be Jewish. Is this pure clannishness — Jewish clannishness, specifically — or is something else going on?

For a long time in the United States, ethnicity was not so much a secret as something that was not generally featured: those whose ethnic origins were not obvious often wished not to emphasize them. Better, it was felt, to be an American, un-hyphenated, than an Italo-, Polish-, Russo-, Greco-, Chinese-, or any other kind of hyphenated American. The hyphen suggested recent immigrant, frequently even more recent working-class, origins, and it felt a bit un-American. Ethnicity was viewed as not a particularly good thing. Hold, then, the hyphen.

Sometime in the 1970s all this changed. The pressure was off, and suddenly it was all right — more than all right — to own up to being Irish-, Polish-, Italian-, Mexican-, Jewish-American. Lay on the hyphens, by all means, and while you're at it, bring out the pasta, burritos, red beans and greens, matzo-ball soup: ethnicity became a badge of authenticity. Coming out of the working class was itself no disgrace — quite the reverse: in many quarters it was a badge of honor.

People under forty may not be aware that fifty years ago there was still strong religious segregation in America. Universities had quotas against Jews and Catholics. Many country clubs would admit neither. (African Americans weren't even in contention for such places.) Whole neighborhoods were known to be "restricted," a euphemism for *Judenrein,* or Jew-clean, arranged through a covenant among neighbors not to sell their houses to Jewish families. At major universities — certainly this was true of the Big Ten schools in the Middle West — fraternities and sororities were strictly segregated among Jews and Gentiles, with some not allowing Catholics, either. University faculties, especially in their English and philosophy departments, avoided hiring Jews. All this brought about a heightened consciousness of one's religious status — and religious and ethnic status were usually connected — a complicated mixture of pride and shame in being what, through the lottery of birth, one was.

From grade school through high school, I grew up in something approaching a sixty-forty Jewish-Gentile demographic distribution in neighborhoods and public schools. In the neighborhood on the Far North Side of Chicago in which my family first lived, most of the non-Jews were Catholics, and this was in a day when the Catholic Church was central to its adherents' lives: for them not to send their kids to Catholic schools, for them to marry non-Catholics, for them to eat meat on Fridays, these were considered radical departures from the norm. As a child, not yet ten, I took Catholicism to be synonymous with Christianity, so pervasive was the Catholic Church in Chicago; no other form of Christianity impinged on my consciousness.

In the second neighborhood of my youth, which was becoming more and more Jewish, Catholics did not seem so dominant. But many Gentiles had fled at the rising number of Jews moving in. Still, I would guess that my classmates were roughly two-thirds Jewish. At the high school I attended, the division between Jews and Gentiles must have been the same, with the Jews representing, sociologically, the ascending lower middle class, and the Gentiles, many of them Swedes and Germans and Irish, mired in the working classes. Social arrangements here were segregated by religion, and it was rare for Gentile and Jewish kids to date one another or to belong to the same clubs. Such integration as there was occurred chiefly on athletic teams.

In both these neighborhoods and at both schools, I had good friends among non-Jews, but most of my closer friends were Jews. In the army I was practically Jew-free (sounds like "Jeffrey" with a goofy accent). Few Jews showed up in my barracks; I chose not to go to Friday night services, where I might meet other Jews. The person I spent the most time with was a Swede, from Oak Park, Illinois. We had both gone to college, thought of ourselves as big-city boys, had in common an ironic sense of humor and skill at ping-pong, but little else.

We were perhaps companions more than friends — that is, if the army hadn't thrown us together, we might never have thought to keep company. Each of us seemed to the other, in the army setting, the closest thing to a friend on offer. After we left the service, he went into the insurance business, and I bought such insurance as I needed from him. He lived a thoroughly suburban existence: married, with two daughters. I would call him from time to time, usually on matters having to do with auto insurance. At longish intervals we would meet for lunch. I learned that he had lost a college-age daughter in a car accident, which gave him an aura of sadness and depth he hadn't previously had for me.

But we were not interested in the same things and, long out of the army, hadn't any subjects to fall back on for conversation. We continued to joke with each other, but the laughter began, at least to me, to seem a little hollow. He was eager to retire, and did, before, I believe, the age of sixty. I learned about his retirement from his insurance office, where, when I once called about a minor claim, a secretary told me that he was no longer there. Fishing had become his thing, and he had acquired a small summer place in Wisconsin where he hoped to fish out his days. Poof — gone.

I fear he looked upon me as a cosmopolitan Jew, though I'm not sure that adjective would have occurred to him. At our rare lunch meetings, when I took him to what I thought the most ordinary restaurants, he found them, I could tell, slightly exotic. His was a mayonnaise-and-white-bread midwestern culture, surrounded by golfers and fishermen. A book-reading — a book-writing, for God's sake — Jew was also exotic to him, I'm sure. I even sensed — and I hope standard Jewish paranoia wasn't kicking in here — a touch of anti-Semitism, in the stray remark he would make suggesting ingrained Jewish business acumen (of which I turn out to have, alas, all too little). From the beginning, it now seems clear, we could go only so far in our relationship with each other, and no farther.

The odd thing is that I can easily imagine — actually, I don't have to imagine — Jews with whom I have as few shared interests. Yet with them more relaxed relationships have been possible, though also not sustainable; but at least walls were broken down more quickly. Interests apart, with other Jews I feel what I can only call a historical commonality. Even among self-hating Jews, this feeling comes through. I once worked for Mortimer J. Adler, who was born a Jew but for many years attended an Episcopal church, and who once instructed a friend of mine who was his office manager not to hire a Jewish girl as his secretary (Adler converted to Catholicism shortly before he died). Around me this man, who identified himself as little as possible as Jewish, would occasionally bring out a Yiddishism or recount stories of his immigrant father. Something about me, apparently, brings out the Jew in people.

I don't take particular pride in feeling a quicker rapport — should it be *rappaport?* — with Jews than with non-Jews. I much prefer to think myself a more universalist character. And some of my best friends, let me quickly add, are not Jews. I should like to be blind to ethnicity, to choose my friends solely on their merits, the kindness of their spirit, the goodness of their hearts. And insofar as I am able, I try to do exactly that. And yet, and yet . . .

A three-way friendship I've always admired, though I know it only from a distance, was that among the poet W. H. Auden, the cultural historian Jacques Barzun, and the literary critic Lionel Trilling. Auden was an Anglican who was openly homosexual; Barzun was French born and without, so far as I know, strong religious affiliation, but quite acceptable in American WASP surroundings; Trilling was ineradicably Jewish, but made a special effort to detach himself from Jewish professional connections (for this reason he refused, as a younger man, to serve on the board of the *Menorah Journal* magazine). What these three men had in common was, of course, great intellectual sophistication and a deep interest in culture. I like to think that this was enough, and more than enough, to sustain a civilized three-way friendship. What I don't know is how close they really were as a triad, especially Barzun's and Trilling's friendship with Auden.

One of my dearest friends is an Irish, New England–bred, Harvard-educated though lower-middle-class-born medical scientist. Despite the differences in our backgrounds, I found our understanding of each other almost immediate and, I believe, perfectly reciprocated. There is nothing I can't say to him that I can say to anyone who is Jewish — except perhaps to mock the Jews, for guilt-free anti-Semitism is one of the secret minor pleasures of being Jewish (as is knocking one's own in any ethnic group). He has proven a friend in every way. We share a view that the world is filled with — sorry for the phrase, but I cannot find another that fits so well — bullshitters, especially in intellectual and scientific life, and that they must be dealt with. I feel a genuine closeness to him; and, what is more, I do not think we would be any closer if he were Jewish or I were not.

And yet I suspect there is something natural about gravitating to one's own people. Greeks I know feel this about fellow Greeks, blacks among blacks (where they can indulge in some truth-telling that would elsewhere pass, I am sure, for pure racism), Poles among Poles, and so on up and down the American ethnic roster. What is a bit unusual, and all the more impressive for its unnaturalness, is when a deep friendship is struck by two people who ostensibly have very little in common — nationality, ethnicity, social class, or intellectual interests — but good faith and good feeling.

Obviously there is comfort in familiarity, something pleasing about knowing that someone has been brought up in a way not all that different from the way you were brought up, has eaten the same kind of food as a child, has been told many of the same wise and dopey stories, has had similar experiences generally. This is part of the comfort — or comfort level, as we nowadays say — that common ethnicity allows.

Living as I do in the same city in which I grew up, I have noticed that many of the boys with whom I went to high school seem, fifty years later, not greatly to have widened their friendships, which are almost all among fellow Jews, many of them old classmates. They belong to the same country clubs, play golf together, meet with one another, wives in tow, on holidays and special occasions. My own circle of friends is greater only because of my line of work. But had I become a physician, lawyer, or businessman and remained in Chicago, doubtless I would be part of this crowd, seeing almost exclusively these same (now old) Jewish boys.

Clannishness has historically been one of the accusations made against Jews. At its most dangerous, that charge was behind the notorious *Protocols of the Elders of Zion,* a paranoid "document" that posited an international Jewish conspiracy to control the world. But Jews themselves came to believe in Jewish clannishness. An old joke has a Jewish man reading the Arab press because it pleases him, while doing so, to read about how powerful and influential the Jews are.

In *The Pity of It All: A History of the Jews in Germany, 1743–1933,* Amos Elon cites the program of a Jewish group formed early in the nineteenth century that set out to reform German Jews by secularizing them, and under the rubric of "Matters in Need of Improvement Among Jews" is noted an item that reads: "The delusion, contrary to law, that it is permissible to cheat non-Jews." Anyone with any knowledge of the sociology of Jewish life knows that Jews are sufficiently disputatious among themselves to make genuine durable clannishness, let alone the *Protocols,* unworkable.

But cliques and clans do not require ethnicity to form. Cliquishness implies exclusion, which is the darker side of friendship. In his novel *Snobs,* Julian Fellowes writes: "The English of all classes, as it happens, are addicted to exclusivity. Leave three Englishmen in a room and they will invent a rule that prevents a fourth joining them." Much of the literature of friendship features it as a one-on-one affair — or, as the sociologists prefer to term it, "dyadic." Add another player or two, forming a web of friendships, and the game can change radically.

Cliques must be one of the earliest forms of social organization going. They set in during childhood, where four or five of the better boy athletes or prettier young girls form a group that implicitly keeps out other kids who are not thought qualified to join their circle. The ins and the outs form the organizing principle of the clique. The older the children get, the clearer the boundaries of in and out are drawn. Sometimes they last a lifetime.

A number of women have told me that young girls are more cliquish than boys — and much crueler in making those not in the clique feel like outsiders. By the time I was in the eighth grade, clubs had formed. Clubs and fraternities and sororities are of course cliquishness organized (as Henry James once called aristocracy "bad manners organized"). These clubs were formed partly on the basis of common interests, but just as much on what were felt to be common social attributes. They were also hierarchical, the hierarchy running from what was considered best to less and less admired. As a boy and young man with sensitive social antennae, my own experience was to get myself into the best of these clubs and then find them disappointing, usually because I had changed and passed on to other interests.

In an excellent essay titled "Community, Society, and the Individual," Yi-Fu Tuan, of the University of Wisconsin, writes about his individuality that "I am a man who identifies with Beethoven's symphonies, Mozart's piano sonatas, certain arias from Peking opera, Tolstoy's *Death of Ivan Ilych,* the aphorisms of Simone Weil, Steven Underhill's photographs, the movie *A.I.: Artificial Intelligence,* my Doty school condominium, kung pao chicken and fried potstickers. The desert landscape, too, is me." Reading that list, I feel that Professor Tuan and I might be able to do business as friends; perhaps I can talk him out of what I feel must be his overvaluation of Simone Weil, and he can explain to me who Steven Underhill is. If we can find a third person — and I feel confident we can — we'd be on our way to having a clique.

At the heart of Professor Tuan's essay is the search for friends to whom one can divulge one's uniqueness, if only because theirs figures to be in many ways similar to one's own. (There's an irony here, of course — a desire to confirm uniqueness by finding it repeated in another.) He cites the friendship of Bertrand Russell and Joseph Conrad, with its immediate sense of connection, especially on the part of Russell, who wrote: "At our very first meeting, we talked with continually increasing intimacy. We seemed to sink through layer after layer of what was superficial, till gradually both reached the central fire.

It was an experience unlike any other that I have known. We looked into each other's eyes half appalled and half intoxicated to find ourselves together in such a region."

Russell's notion of a "central fire" suggests something communal, fit for more than two: a community of friends. Odd that Bertrand Russell should have felt this with Joseph Conrad, for the two men, at least in their politics, were not merely different but, had each trotted out his political views, strongly opposed: Russell holding out endless hope for human beings when properly organized (as he came at one point to think that the Soviet Union was), and Conrad feeling that men and women were at bottom alone in the world (which didn't, it needs to be added, stop him from longing for friendship).

The central fire, then, is something beyond and deeper than mere agreement. It is a place where one can receive kindness, understanding, solace, patient attention, and respect for one's point of view, and all this because of an underlying but never spoken sense that everyone around that central fire, or in the community, knows that he and she are all in the same struggle together.

Community is a concept with a long history. It suggests life at a level less complex than that of a full-blown society, a cohesive group within the larger society where a cooperative spirit reigns and each person feels the glow of good feeling and concern for everyone else. Utopian movements hold out the promise of universal community; the rarity of real community is what makes these movements utopian. Under the once promised Communist "dictatorship of the proletariat," full-time, full-scale community was the goal. I once heard a man sympathetic to the Soviet Union say that he never watches movies on videotape or DVD because he loses "the sense of community" that going to the movies provides. This, I would say, is pushing it.

The word "community" took a beating some years ago through vast overuse. During this time one heard lots about the "black community," the "Jewish community," the "gay community," the "artistic community," and even, sadly, the "homeless community." Communities cannot be so large, so differentiated within themselves—blacks, Jews, gays, and artists are sufficiently divided among themselves to render talk of them as true communities meaningless. Potential voting blocs they may be; communities, not even close. No one has ever laid down a limitation in number for a true community, but I would set the number at thirty, at the outside thirty-five people. More than that and the intensity of feeling, and with it the intensity of common delight, dissipates.

Most of us, I suspect, have at one time or another been members of true communities. The most typical may be membership on athletic teams, especially when the team is doing well. In my own case, the sense of community, when I have experienced it, has been fairly short-lived. I felt I belonged to the community formed by the twenty-five or so men in my platoon during the difficult weeks of basic training in the army. I felt it earlier among my fellow fraternity pledges during a semester at the University of Illinois, though I couldn't feel anything like it for the full fraternity, and moved out soon after having become a member. Interestingly, in both cases, the army and the fraternity pledgeship, I was living full-time and at close quarters with members of these groups.

I've never felt anything similar for a political community—quite the reverse: when I find myself in a room with people whom I can count on to share (roughly) my own political views, my first thought is that perhaps these views are flawed and I ought to rethink them. Academics used to speak of a "community of scholars," but in a thirty-year teaching career, I have never felt anything like the warmth of Bertrand Russell's central fire at a university. Perhaps people with narrow special interests—stamp collectors, historians of eighteenth-century medicine, orchid growers—feel themselves seated at the fire. Among my fellow writers, alas, I have never felt anything closer than the real but less than communal pleasure of talking shop.

But on those occasions, however brief, when I have felt myself part of a community, the feeling was enormously satisfying. The feeling is one of belonging. You look at the others seated around the central fire and feel with equal confidence that you would do almost anything for these people, as they would do almost anything for you. As a member of a community, you feel you have lost yourself, however temporarily, in something larger, of which you are nonetheless an important part. To be part of a true community is to experience collective friendship, with the associated feelings of mutuality and reciprocity that are normally available only between two people. It's a grand, grand feeling, and all the grander for its rarity.

# 14

◇

## *Talking the Talk*

THE SUBJECT OF FRIENDSHIP invokes much discourse about loyalty, trust, intimacy, confession, soulfulness, betrayal, and other large and highflying matters. But as I remarked earlier, in most friendships many of these things are never, even after decades, called into play. And when they are, often they are called in only briefly: the friend either comes through or he doesn't, and then it's back to business as usual; often, even if he doesn't come through, the friendship manages to survive and stay intact. Friendship shouldn't entail a checklist of virtues that a person has to pass to become one's friend. Besides, once one has set up such a list, there is the distinct possibility that one cannot oneself measure up to it.

At the heart of most friendships is something much simpler: talk and, going on beneath the talk, understanding, preferably easy, immediate understanding. One may fish, golf, quilt, or play bridge with a friend, one may or may not share his or her opinions, one may have many or few interests in common, but what most friends do with one another much of the time is talk. The style of talk in good part sets the tone of one's friendship. One might have, with different people, bantering talk, or challenging talk, or artfully conveyed subtle talk, or amusingly combative talk, or slightly-dull-but-still-comforting-because-familiar talk. Certain friendships, based almost entirely on longevity, may call for very little talk. But above all, in one's talk with friends one seeks relaxed enjoyment. Friendship, when it goes well, is harmony played on the instrument of conversation.

"The truth is, that in our habitual intercourse with others, we much oftener require to be amused than assisted," William Hazlitt remarks in his essay "Characteristics." "We consider less, therefore, what a person with whom we are intimate is ready to do for us in critical emergencies, than what he has to say on ordinary occasions." Hazlitt nails the point precisely: the chief pleasure of friendship comes about through talk.

The best philosophical explanation for this comes from another, much-later-born Englishman, the political philosopher Michael Oakeshott, who, in a few pertinent paragraphs in his *Rationalism in Politics and Other Essays,* makes the simple yet crucial distinction that friendship is at bottom not instrumental but dramatic. In friendship, Oakeshott holds, "attachment springs from an intimation of familiarity and subsists in a mutual sharing of personalities. To go on changing one's butcher until one gets the meat one likes, to go on educating one's agent until he does what is required of him, is conduct not inappropriate to the relationship concerned; but to exchange friends because they do not behave as we expected and refuse to be educated to our requirements is the conduct of a man who has altogether mistaken the character of friendship. Friends are not concerned with what might be made of one another, but only with the enjoyment of one another, and the condition of this enjoyment is a ready acceptance of what is and the absence of any desire to change or to improve."

Elsewhere Oakeshott writes: "A friend is not someone one trusts to behave in a certain manner, who has certain useful qualities, who holds acceptable opinions; he is someone who evokes interest, delight, unreasoning loyalty, and who (almost) engages contemplative imagination." You like your friends, in other words, for what they are and not for their use to you, however useful some of them may also, on unexpected occasions, turn out to be. You like them, too, because you can talk comfortably with them.

I recently had dinner at a Chinese restaurant on the North Side of Chicago with two longtime male friends. We began with that lingua franca of American men, sports talk. The Cubs had earlier in the day lost a twelve-inning game that would help take them out of postseason play, and we eased into our conversation by analyzing, in a mildly grumbling way, the team's inadequacies. We've had this discussion before, in other years and with other Cubs teams, with different personnel involved and in different settings. But it's all right among friends of long standing: a bit of redundancy is tolerable; it's even comforting to go over this only slightly changed ground one more time. Each of us contributes what small insights he has on the subject. None of us is disputatious; there are no arguments; a common spirit of mature, humorous resignation reigns.

I brought along a paperback copy of Walter Jackson Bate's *Samuel Johnson* for one of these two friends of mine. I remark to the other, who is in publishing, that I didn't bring him a book, for everyone knows that editors don't have time for reading. This leads my friend to talk a little about the publishing business, how difficult it has become, the oppressive pall cast on small firms such as his own by the big chain bookstores. I've heard this before, too, though this time out my friend adds a few new twists.

Which leads us into anecdotes about a wild, zany Chicago bookseller, now retired, who has a nervous disorder that causes him to stammer — a stammer that he suppresses by drinking a martini or two, which causes him to act outrageously. Only two of us have such anecdotes, I and my friend in publishing; the third friend has long been in the mortgage business, though he reads serious books and has an abiding appreciation of the oddities of character. We fill him in on details he figures to be unaware of about the bookseller. He is a good listener. So is my other friend. I hope I am too, though calling oneself a good listener is always dangerous, like declaring oneself generous, a great lover, a completely honorable person — these are determinations for others to make.

I bring up having had lunch with a man of some local celebrity as a jazz pianist and vibraphonist (he is sometimes mentioned in lists that include Lionel Hampton), who went to high school with me and my friend in the mortgage business. This requires supplying some background information to our friend in publishing. The musician I lunched with had a tough adolescence; he was nerdy and unkempt and two years ahead of himself in school. Socially, ours was a grueling school, hard on anyone unable to meet the brutal tests of conformity in strict force there.

Which leads the three of us into a discussion of our days as college fraternity men and the comedy of standards of superficiality and what passed for elegance then. Two of us had spent a year in fraternities at the University of Illinois; my friend in publishing had put in four years at Zeta Beta Tau at the University of Missouri. He tells a story of a boy who made the fatal error of wearing a suede belt and suede shoes to a dance, for which sin, through the remainder of his days, he was known as Felt Belt Goldstein (though I recall only the epithet, not his actual last name).

We somehow drift into talk of the current (2004) presidential race, and agree on the thorough inadequacy of both incumbent and challenger. My friend in the mortgage business is perhaps more indifferent to politics than anyone I know; it is one of the many reasons I like him. My friend in publishing takes more interest in these things, but is as far from being fanatical about them as possible: he is instead earnest, his earnestness seasoned with the proper amount of dubiety and humor. We don't stay on this subject for very long. None of the three of us is looking for an argument that would end in his victory. Unlike much male-to-male talk, no note of even mild aggressiveness erupts throughout the lunch.

After the check and the almond and fortune cookies arrive, we linger before dividing the bill. I tell a joke that gets a good response. Now that I recall the lunch, I think I did more talking than my two friends. I hope I didn't dominate in any way, for I have become conscious in recent years of the danger of becoming a gasbag, someone who has acquired too many jokes and too large a repertoire of anecdotes, and I am consequently fearful of resembling the man who returns from a party to report to his wife that if it hadn't been for his own brilliant talk, he would have been bored blue.

Much general jokiness pervaded our two-and-a-half-hour meeting. Out on the street, we shake hands, pledging to get together again before long. We probably shall not meet again as a trio for seven or eight months, possibly longer. Each of us walks off in a different direction. I get into my car thinking that, though nothing significant or new had been said and nothing whatsoever had been accomplished, it was nonetheless a successful meeting, given over to the simple pleasures of friendship. I really like these guys, I tell myself; I'm glad they are my friends.

Not all talk among friends is as easy for me as this lunch meeting. Some talk is more exciting, some more droll, some a bit dull, which is all right too, since on occasion the magic of friendship isn't there, even with longtime and beloved friends.

The crux of conversation in friendship is the willingness to listen. "Being listened to is one of the few aphrodisiacs left," according to a writer in *Ms.* magazine. Not for nothing does the item come from *Ms.*, for women may feel the need to be listened to more than men. I have heard the sight, so often on view in restaurants and bars, of a man leaning in and talking intensely to a woman, described as "the missionary position." This is amusing but also sad in its accuracy. Finding people who listen is often quite as difficult among men, too.

Good listeners may be as rare, perhaps rarer, than good talkers. Max Beerbohm noted of the English critic Desmond MacCarthy that his voice contained an "endearing intimacy"; his talk was a form of "chamber music," for McCarthy was especially adept at bringing other people into the conversation, and he was also "a great user of that beguiling phrase, 'And tell me.'"

Most of us, in our friendships, seem to want more to tell than to be told. We see, we use, friends as an audience — and friends in their turn often do the same with us. Many conversations aren't really conversations at all, but merely alternating monologues. Was it Nora Ephron who said that there is no listening, only waiting — waiting, of course, to do one's own talking?

Winston Churchill, that most brilliant of talkers, is said to have been a poor listener; Goethe, himself a dab hand at talk, had the reputation of being a careful listener.

To turn briefly to stereotypes, women were once thought too talkative, the word for which was "gabby," and in the old movies certain second-banana female stars (Billie Burke, Spring Byington) played the flibbertigibbet role amusingly. Men, in the same line of stereotyping, are thought to be laconic. The Hemingway heroes are men of few words; in the *noir* movies of the late 1930s and 1940s, economy of speech is also the rule: think Bogart, or of the dialogue supplied for him by Raymond Chandler and Dashiell Hammett. Westerns were even less talky: Jimmy Stewart, John Wayne, and Henry Fonda made plain that their pistols did their talking for them, blazing six-guns firing blanks, of course, and when the stars opened their mouths to speak, blank, too, was most of the talk they emitted.

In a good conversation among friends attentiveness must not only be a key element but must also be reciprocal. I recently attended a dinner at which four of the people were women, three men. The most intelligent person in the room was a man, and he, generally full of interesting and provocative information (please be assured, he isn't the author of this book), was crowded out by the stale jokes and professional complaints of one of the other men in the room (still not me). A sadly wasted evening, I thought.

M.F.K. Fisher, the writer on food, sets out what she deems a perfect sextet of dinner guests under the assumption that food and talk go together: "The six should be capable of decent social behavior: that is, no two of them should be so much in love as to bore the others, nor at the opposite extreme should they be carrying on any sexual or professional feud which could poison the plates all must eat from. A good combination would be one married couple, for warm composure; one less firmly established, to add a note of investigation to the talk; and two strangers of either sex, upon whom the better acquainted could sharpen their questioning wit."

What might be the perfect friendship equivalent of such a table? My own setting would call for three men and three women, all of whom like one another a lot; whether they are married or not doesn't much matter. A roughly equal regard for the talents, intelligence, and good humor of everyone at the table must reign. In the conversation among them, explanation would be allowed, condescension placed out of bounds. All that would be predictable among the six is their decency; banter would be permitted, but the spirit of one-upmanship, let alone of the caustic putdown, would be *verboten*. All would have enough confidence in their own opinions not to need to have them confirmed by everyone else in the room, though differing opinions — on politics, artistic taste, religion — might add a touch of garlic to the proceedings. But the point of view of each guest would be much more important than his or her mere opinions. Each would have an underlying, though never a heavy or otherwise dampening, seriousness.

This seriousness would not preclude a taste for the sweet pleasantries of small talk. *Gravitas* is fine in its place, but then so is *levitas,* which I, for one, require to sustain not only my friendships but my own well-being. *Levitas,* or lightness of spirit, often appears in the guise of small talk, which over the years has taken a bad rap. The phrase "small talk" is close to an automatic pejorative. "Look," some people say, "let's skip the small talk." Or: "My meeting with her was a complete flop; we never got beyond small talk." Clearly not a good thing, small talk; something to be got out of the way, hurried past, best to have nothing to do with in the first place.

I happen to like small talk. Eliminate a few small-talk standbys — the weather, say, or the traffic — and I find it in and of itself a splendid thing. Given a choice, I almost always prefer small to big talk. I don't long to sit around with friends and discuss whether God may be said to exist after the Holocaust. Or if another close national election might be the death knell for the Electoral College. Nor do I long to hear discussions about abortion in any of its aspects.

If I were to hear any of these subjects broached as I was about to walk into a room, I would turn around and depart smartly. I should much prefer to enter a room where a conversation is going on in which someone claims that it is impossible for an American to speak French well, or avers that the sizing of American clothes has lost all standardization, or asks if it's true that John F. Kennedy wasn't merely a skirt chaser but had an actual sex addiction. Now these I take to be subjects that have the potential to inspire wit, amusing anecdotes, oddly angled points of view—to make, in short, for unpredictable and charming conversation among friends or recent acquaintances. And, as a bonus, they might lead interestingly into other subjects—perhaps, who knows, some of them approaching big talk, though not, let us hope, of a lumpish kind.

Although people regularly insist that they have no small talk—thereby, by indirection, postulating their large-mindedness—the truth is that some people are incapable of reaping the pleasures of such talk. Those who talk for victory are disqualified; so, too, are those who find themselves crushed when their opinions aren't duplicated by those of everyone else in the room; and one must include those well into what I call their anecdotage, that branch of nonlisteners who are only looking for ways to insert their eight or ten stale stories into the conversation, no matter the actual subject up for discussion.

Maybe the best way to avoid charmless talk is to place too much importance on one's own opinions—on food, movies, child-rearing, politics, religion, and a few other ill-chosen subjects. A person's opinions are perhaps the least important thing about him. Besides, everyone surely has had the experience of finding someone who holds most of one's own opinions and yet discovers that that person is nonetheless a terminal bore; or, conversely, meets someone whose opinions are strikingly different from one's own and finds her captivatingly interesting.

The best talkers are those who are devoted to keeping the conversation going. These same people frequently turn out also to be the best listeners. They view sociability as a form of musical composition—a string quartet or octet of the Baroque, perhaps. In their understanding of a good conversation, talk ought, like a winning musical composition, to have melody, harmony, and development; it ought also to take gently surprising turns and twists and end with everyone who has taken part glowing with pleasure and, as the conclusion nears, wanting more. Not easily achieved, such conversation, yet when it does come about, how light and free and fine life appears. And how richly rewarding friendship seems.

Naturally, not all talk in friendship can be charming. Sometimes a plunge into deeper waters cannot be eluded. I recently had lunch with a friend whom I meet roughly once a year. We have known each other for twenty-five years. He knows a few foreign languages and was educated in classics. Our conversations in the past were largely persiflage, amusing (to me at least) chat, heavy on the irony, light on the dreary, only rarely lapsing, and then obliquely, into the depths.

He waited until fifty to marry, and had three children soon thereafter. And then he was struck by what may well be the central sadness of his life: his younger (than he) wife turned out to be bipolar, with the awful trimmings that illness brings with it, heavy drinking and paranoid fantasies among them. Our conversations are now more and more given over to the difficulties of his days as a father who must do everything he can, with limited financial resources, to save his three daughters from a mother gripped by manic depression.

As it happens, I have a relative, a man, in the same condition as my friend, and I can at least contribute what little I know, through my having spoken a great deal about his situation with this relative. The experience has — no surprise here — taken much of the jauntiness from my friend: his *gravitas-levitas* balance has shifted considerably. And yet I find him more attractive now. His troubles, in their significance — the lives of three children, after all, are at stake — have changed everything, even his appearance. He now has the look of what these troubles have made him: that of a man who has been put through a few of life's more exquisite tortures, but also, as a result, the look of a man of character.

At our last conversation, at a Greek restaurant in Chicago, he told me how much he has come to appreciate his now eighty-four-year-old father. To have had a parent of steadiness, who stayed on the job without being in any way smothering in his attentions, who kept up a vein of good humor without losing any of his authority, seems to him today a piece of skillful fathering and, for him as the recipient of such skill, a piece of great good luck. As he talked further, I recognized, too, that he is a man of whom his father would, I think, be proud. Our lunches have less laughter, yet I find I now enjoy his company more.

The ideal conversation among friends is, I suppose, for many modeled on the college bull session. I'm not thinking of bull sessions of the formal, fraternity or sorority kind, where a fairly large group of young men or women get together to straighten one another out on this or that odd or unacceptable bit of social behavior. What I am thinking of are those magical nights where two, at the outside three, friends get together to talk in a let-your-hair-down, shoes-off way about their dreams and fears.

I cannot remember ever taking part in such sessions, and when I ask myself why, I think it must have to do with the odd line of work, writing, that I determined to do in my late adolescence. To be nineteen or twenty and tell friends that you want to be a writer sounded empty and at the same time pretentious, even fantastical. My dreams (to be a serious writer) and fears (to fail abysmally at it) were too unreal and scarifying to discuss with anyone, my parents included. Instead I merely wrote, began to publish, and looked up one day and — lo! — discovered I was a writer, with all the delights and detractions pertaining thereto. Then, when it was no longer a dream but a reality, there was no need for bull sessions to talk about it.

At what point in life does one stop talking to friends about one's dreams? I believe I may have passed it; in my mid-sixties, dream time is over. Such dreams as I have are for my grandchildren, and these are about their arriving through life's dangerous waters into safe harbor. My fears are too obvious to require discussion: departing the planet ahead of schedule, also known as death. More and more, as I grow older, I spend time listening to younger people tell me about their dreams and fears. "Tell me," I used to say when meeting students about to graduate, "about your plans for your brilliant career."

But the most rewarding talk for me nowadays is with friends settled in life, and not displeased with where it has landed them. I meet with A roughly once a month. He was a local bookseller who also taught social science at a community college. He is eight or so years older than I, grew up in a Yiddish-speaking household, is well married, the father of four children. "You are rich," Henry James has a character in *The Portrait of a Lady* say, "when you can meet the demands of your imagination." By this measure, A is rich. The last time we were together he told me that he had achieved almost everything he always wanted: he ran a bookstore, was a community college teacher, made money through investing; all that was missing, he said, was that he would also have liked to run a successful restaurant.

What makes A unusual is his contentment in life. Despite his living with some of the same difficulties that in one form or another confront us all, this contentment seems near complete. Some while ago he made the sound decision to savor every aspect of his life, from his morning coffee to the music he plays on his superior sound system to the view outside his study windows to every morsel of food he puts in his mouth. This decision has kept him youthful-looking at seventy-eight, and still ardent for life, of which he wants lots more.

Although we do not go back that far — I first met A while frequenting his bookstore — only in the past five or six years have we become closer friends. Our talk has a fairly high level of candor. Perhaps the main difference between us is his social-science and my literary training and outlook. He tends to look for the meaty generalization, I for the exception that proves no rule. Never in therapy himself, he has seen successful therapy applied to members of his family; and, in fact, one of his daughters is a therapist. He is quicker than I to say what might be troubling him about a friendship; he is also more easily put off by philistinism than I.

At our last meeting, over coffee, late on a Monday morning, we talked about a notion that came up in connection with an essay I had not long before written about the novelist Isaac Bashevis Singer. This had to do with what I took to be the drama that each of us carries around in his head of how the world works and his or her own role in it. I had in mind the drama of acquiring power, or fame, or wealth, or knowledge, possibly all of these together; the drama of turning one's back on the great world to become a superior father/mother, husband/wife, son/daughter; the drama of alienation, or finding the world foolish in not recognizing one for one's subtle but quite real talents.

Ever the social scientist, A pressed me to fill out the notion sufficiently so that it might attain the dignity of an idea. I babbled on a fair amount, without, I think, much success. Somehow the notion of personal drama got mixed up with role-playing, a much simpler thing and not at all what I had in mind. Later that day, he sent me a lengthy e-mail summarizing our conversation on this point — though we talked about other things during our meeting — and the next day he sent me two further e-mails, adding yet more. Good stuff, too. But I realize, as I think about A, that one of the things I value in him is his passion. He has a warmer nature than mine, and I sometimes feel that I do not respond to him as fully as he might wish.

I thought again of Henry James's aphorism about one's being rich when one can meet the demands of one's imagination when I had a lunch date with two figures from my boyhood days whom I hadn't seen in fifty years. They are suburban, partners in an insurance business; each has had one marriage, in which he seems content. They are grandfathers now, and well settled in that role. They have reconnected with me through my writing. One of them reads a magazine in which my writing appears regularly, and he took it upon himself to get in touch with me; I suggested we meet for lunch, and now here we are.

The conversation picks up as if we had seen one another last month and not half a century ago. This is because we come from the same place: grew up with the same assumptions, manners, inflections in our speech. The poet August Kleinzahler, in a memoir called "My Girls," has formulated the experience I feel with these two men, and they with me, when he writes about talking with a boyhood pal from New Jersey: "He is from the neighborhood, a place that no longer exists except in memory. Those of us from the neighborhood pass among others in this world, like the mendicants who carried with them the record of classical learning through the drear, cobbled passageways of the Dark Ages. Even if we don't recognize one another or recognize the face, we are able to spot one another, at cross-walks, shopping plazas, train platforms. A look suffices. Nothing needs to be spoken."

I don't know for how long they have been partners, but in one respect they remind me, these two men now in late middle age, of an old married couple. Each has probably heard all the other's anecdotes many times over, and when one or the other unsheathes one for me, the other waits patiently until it is time for him to unsheathe his. The anecdotes are all fresh to me, of course, and of interest, since most of them have to do with people I knew in my late adolescence, about many of whom they brought me up to date. The flow of talk through a ninety-minute lunch was easy, insignificant, and pleasing.

An aura of good feeling pervades out on the sidewalk in front of the restaurant, where we shake hands. I thank them for buying my lunch. We tell one another that it's been great; and in fact it has been pretty damn nice. We also tell one another we must arrange to meet again soon. My guess is that we probably shan't, but somehow that's all right, too.

The next day I have lunch with a former student, now in his early forties, who lives in Minneapolis and works for a consulting firm that requires him to do a lot of traveling—often four days every week, much more than he, with a wife and a two-year-old daughter at home, likes. We don't meet often—perhaps once a year, and sometimes a few years go by without our meeting—but whenever we do meet I am freshly charmed to see how increasingly impressive he has become. This time I note a slight growth of gray hair at his temples.

Over lunch we talk a fair amount about baseball. He is a life-time Boston Red Sox fan, and that evening the Red Sox are playing the Yankees in the seventh game of the playoffs to determine who will go to the World Series (which, as history now records, the Red Sox did). When I was editing a magazine, he wrote a solid article for me on the Red Sox outfielder Carl Yastrzemski, the great Yaz, that showed the ballplayer's possession of the unusual combination of talent, hard work, and character, which the author of the article himself now seems well on his way to acquiring.

We talk about his family. He has had a daughter late enough in life to appreciate what a miracle it all is. We talk about real estate and the wild prices of houses. We talk about his parents, who are close to my age, their health and temperamental condition. We talk about his work, about the prospect of going into business for himself. We do not run out of subjects or come close to doing so. After lunch we walk back to my apartment; at the entrance to the building, we shake hands. I tell him how much I enjoyed our meeting, and that I hope we can have many more in the years ahead. As he walks off to his car, I think this was a very good kid now become an impressive man.

Variety is the keynote of the friendships I have described in this chapter. None is, in Michael Oakeshott's sense, "instrumental." I am friends with the people I have described, and they with me, because, with varying degrees of affection, we enjoy one another's company, which really means we take pleasure in our talk, schmooze, rattling on. "This is the happiest conversation," said Samuel Johnson, "where there is no competition, no vanity, but a calm interchange of sentiments." The good doctor, once again, gets it bang-on right.

# 15

❖

## *Techno-Friendships*

Leave a message after the beep.

—POPULAR TWENTY-FIRST-CENTURY SAYING

WHEN I WAS A BOY, I recall the not infrequent occasions when, sitting home with my parents at seven-thirty or eight at night, the doorbell would ring and they would have an unexpected visit from friends. No plans for the visit had been made, no telephone query beforehand was given, just that slightly alarming ring of the doorbell. These friends — I can think of three different couples who did this fairly often — usually brought a pint of ice cream or a bit of pastry, my mother made coffee, and they would sit and talk for a few hours. I suspect my parents could have done just as well without such visits, but I don't remember their complaining about them, even though the doorbell would sometimes catch my father already in his pajamas, out of which he'd quickly change back into his trousers and shirt.

This almost never happens to my wife and me. I do have one friend who sometimes, during the day, will ring my bell unannounced and come up for an hour or so of talk; it is a sign of our good feeling for each other that he knows he can do this. Everyone else calls first, and I do the same when visiting others. In fact, to put my full absence of spontaneity in these matters out into the open, I prefer a couple of days' notice before people visit.

Two possibilities here: one is that the problem is personal, my being unbearably closed-shop in the sociability department, a man with the dry little soul of a hermit; the other is that something has changed in the culture at large. I favor the latter explanation, naturally. What has happened, I think, is that the telephone has become a socially more revolutionary machine than anyone, fifty or even thirty years ago, might have imagined (and I'm not speaking here of the cell phone, with all its subsidiary functions). When I was a kid, the telephone was viewed pretty much as an instrument, or, a touch more precisely, an instrumentality. Conveying messages, setting up appointments, checking in briefly — these were its chief uses. Even those who grew up in relatively easy financial circumstances will recall the speed with which one was expected to talk when making a long-distance call: the three-minute-and-no-more-long-distance telephone call was in those days like the four-minute mile: a record to which everyone aspired.

Rare were the families who had more than one phone in their house or apartment. Less well-off people might have had a phone in the hallway, to be shared among all the tenants in a building. To save on the bill, or sometimes owing to technical limitations in small towns or suburbs, some people also had what were called party lines — party as opposed to private — another shared arrangement in which several families used the same telephone line. Standard jokes were made about busybodies spending their days secretly listening in on party lines to get their fill of local news, fodder for gossip.

The telephone, a bit of a miracle to begin with, was nowhere near so much a part of life as it has become. Soon enough people acquired second phones, then phone lines for their children (older readers will recall the advent of the small, pastel-colored Princess phone, the perfect gift for a spoiled daughter), then the phone required for the at-home fax machine and to get on-line with a modem, and finally the cell phone, owned by a majority of Americans, some of whom would sooner leave home without their wallet or purse or esophagus.

The effect of the pervasiveness of the telephone and all its assorted devices and of e-mail (about which more presently) on friendship has been considerable, if not radical. For starters, reasonably (also unreasonably) lengthy phone conversations meant that one could maintain friendships without actually seeing friends for long periods. Some friendships could indeed be conducted almost wholly by phone (or, now, by e-mail or instant messaging).

Many people might deplore this; these would be people who tend to be slightly Luddite, some of them without their knowing or acknowledging it. Others would argue that no meeting among people who call themselves friends is a true meeting unless handshakes, hugs, or kisses are involved. The flesh must be not only seen but pressed, if only to gain the full nuances of a conversation through noting expressions and body language. Then, too, without tête-à-tête meetings, one loses all of the auxiliary pleasures of friendship — breaking bread together, watching the reactions to one's jokes, looking into each other's eyes — that, thus far at least, cannot be fully achieved through one or another kind of electronic device.

And yet technology has indisputably altered the quality of many friendships. In my own social life, I suspect that I spend as much time on the phone with friends as in actual meetings with them. Whole mornings or afternoons have drifted away from me in telephone talk with friends. Thirty or forty minutes spent on a single phone call with certain friends is not that long for me — at any rate, it does not seem that long when it is passing by. I sometimes get two or three such calls in a single day. When it happens, I feel stupid for tossing away the better part of a morning or afternoon. But it happens, and while it is happening I am hugely enjoying myself.

I have a few friendships that, without the telephone, probably wouldn't exist. I speak at irregular intervals with a friend from New York whom I've known for twenty years in whose presence I have been only three times, and on only two of these occasions were we alone together. He is unmarried, ten or so years younger than I, a literary man. We talk almost exclusively about our common business, which is lit biz. We gas away about other writers, about difficult and pleasant experiences we've had with editors, about deals forged and forgone. We talk about fees with some candor, and about such intellectual notions, inchoate and well formulated, that we have formed or met with in our respective reading. We often start out by promising each other that this time our call will be short; but it seldom runs to less than half an hour and often runs well over that. It's made all the pleasanter by the element of surprise: neither of us knows when he might expect a call from the other. It's the telephone equivalent of my parents' receiving unexpected visits from friends, except in this instance I don't have to put up coffee or, like my father, to change from pajamas back into street clothes.

I have been in New York scores of times without calling this friend, much as I enjoy his talk, much as I like him. The reason might be that we are more comfortable with each other over the phone than in person, though our few meetings have been genial enough. It may even be that if we lived in the same city, we wouldn't be friends at all; we might begin to see each other on a regular basis, and such regularity could bring on boredom. Friendships, as I trust readers who have gotten this far in the book will have noted, can be wildly complex things.

Another friend living in New York, with whom I have been dealing for nearly forty years — he is the editor of a magazine to which I have been a contributor over that period — is also someone I have spent more time on the phone with than in person. We hold lots of views in common; we have grown older together, though I am a few years older than he. We both have memories of a time when intellectuals seemed both more comical and impressive than they do now. He is smart, learned, funny. He also encourages the madcap in me, which is very agreeable; in phone conversations with him I find myself saying goofily comic things. After dealing with each other for so long, we know each other's moves as if we were an old vaudeville team.

I have had other friendships develop out of professional relationships, but none is as long-standing or as satisfying as this one. We've had flare-ups, usually over his desire to rework more radically than I wish something I've written for his magazine. But the flare-ups, on both our sides, preclude go-to-the-mat struggles in which our friendship is at stake. It never is; I don't want it ever to be. I would miss those calls that begin with his secretary — there have eight or ten of them over the years — saying, "Mr. Epstein, will you hold for Mr. K?" If I lived in New York, I should doubtless see more of him. But that we don't see each other for long stretches of time seems all right, too. Meanwhile, always with pleasing anticipation, I hold for Mr. K.

As I write about these two friendships, both of them conducted largely over the telephone, it occurs to me that I am making them sound a bit like the friendship equivalent of phone sex. They are not, of course, anything like the same, at least insofar as I understand phone sex, but friendships conducted for the most part over the phone are not only a reasonable substitute when regular personal meetings aren't possible; but they can have their own, quite different, yet appealing quality.

Proust once said that he didn't much care for the analogy of a book to a friend. He thought a book was better than a friend, because you could shut it — and be shut of it — when you wished, which one can't always do with a friend. With caller ID added to one's telephone service one can, in effect, turn off the lights and sit in the dark until the visitor goes away (a matter of a mere four or five rings of the phone), or, to use Proust's analogy, never "open" the friend to begin with. Screening calls allows one to have conversation with one's friends when one is ready for it. Thank you once again, technology.

Voice mail, too, deserves the thanks of those among us who like conversations with friends on our own terms, or at least at our own chosen times. I have some friends with whom no phone conversation has ever been under twenty minutes; I have other (not very dear) friends whom I'd prefer not to hear from at all. While I don't say, in the words of W. C. Fields, "On second thought, screw 'em," I do say, on first thought, screen 'em — and, let me admit straight out, I sometimes do so without the least twinge of bad conscience.

I also sometimes find myself using voice mail — how should I say? — defensively. I need to make a call to an acquaintance or a friend with whom I don't wish to spend time jabbering on the phone. So I wait until I'm certain he or she is away from the phone and leave my message on voice mail. Fantastico! The English historian R. H. Tawney, author of *Religion and the Rise of Capitalism,* when asked if he noted any progress in his lifetime, is supposed to have replied: "Yes, in the deportment of dogs. Dogs seem much better behaved today than they were when I was a boy." Dogs seem about the same in their deportment to me, but subtle changes in the use of the telephone such as I've just described I count as real progress.

Computer technology, via the Internet, has of course widened and changed the nature of many friendships. People have long used computerized dating services. One such service, called Friendster, has turned into a networking facility for connecting like-minded people, by providing photographs and minibiographies of themselves: a matchmaking, in effect, of friends. Something like four million people were registered at Friendster at last count, most in their twenties and thirties, many overseas, a large number of these Asians. An academic named Danah Boyd, who both uses and studies Friendster, claims that it represents a basic change in the nature of friendship: "Not a mimicry of a change," she says, "it's a total change." I'm not so sure, but a phenomenon such as Friendster does speak to the vast loneliness in the world.

At a lower level of technology, I find myself delighted with e-mail. E-mail has its critics — some say, among other things, that it destroys careful prose composition, others that it has become as much a burden as a convenience — but from the standpoint of friendship it, too, strikes me as a happy invention. Certainly e-mail is a great advance over what used to be called pen pals, which in olden days involved two correspondents, often from different countries, assigned to write to each other, usually beginning in grade school. The advance e-mail represents, of course, is that of quick response. With e-mail one can get directly back to one's correspondents with further queries, responses, addenda. Instant messaging is not something I do, but this makes the response aspect of things even more immediate.

Apart from its speed, e-mail is a great protector against telephone abusers, among whom, for reasons given above, I have to count myself. Before e-mail, I might call a friend to check on a date for a meeting or have him tell me the location of a restaurant or shop, and then, one thing leading to another, stay on the phone for half an hour or more telling jokes, bringing up recent occurrences in either of our lives, or mentioning a mutual friend whom one or the other of us has recently seen. Some people might say, Ah, but such dalliances on the phone or (better) in person are among the true delights in life. Why clip them short? Because of time, because however extensive one's friendships, they mustn't be permitted to dominate one's life, however pleasurable. Such is my puritanical judgment on the matter.

The other advantage of e-mail for me is that I receive a great deal more e-mail from readers than I formerly did letters. The ease of e-mail, the fact that one needs no stamp or mailbox nor has to make obeisance to the formality required by a full-blown letter, encourages readers to send responses to my various scribblings. The number of such e-mails as I receive is not staggering, and any writer who says he would prefer not to be bothered with the responses of his readers at all deserves to have his fingers sewn together, but they must amount to four hundred or so a year. Except for the (very rare) insane or madly ticked-off e-mail I receive, I try to answer it all, some of it laconically, most at modest length.

Many of the people who send me e-mail about things I write seem very attractive, and not merely those who write to compliment me on this or that piece of writing. Several are my contemporaries; a number are younger people asking advice about their own writing; more than a few remark on things they find in my writing that have analogues in their own lives. Very pleasing it is to receive such generous responses to things I write, and without e-mail I doubt, as I say, I should receive a tenth as much communication from readers as I now do.

I also have some (almost regular) e-mail correspondents: a humanities librarian from a university in Michigan; a retired, cultivated reader in North Carolina; a bond salesman in Chicago; a corrector of factual mistakes in my and everyone else's writing in intellectual journals who lives in Maryland; a sharp academic woman from I don't know where; a photographer from San Francisco; a generous culture tout from Palo Alto who sends me jokes and recommends movies and PBS-ish programs I ought to be on the outlook for. I am on a first-name basis with a few of them, on a Mr. and Ms. basis with the rest. With the exception only of the man from Palo Alto and the photographer from San Francisco and the librarian from Michigan, I've not met them.

E-mail has also allowed me to keep in better touch with a few friends I much value who live in Europe — one in France and two in England. We do a bit of business with one another; we pass along jokes and bits of gossip. With two of these three men I sometimes exchange stories and essays we have written. One of the three I've never met but have been reading for thirty or more years, and the rapport between us was immediate. The lovely convenience of it, all made possible by this miraculous invention called e-mail, is a blessed thing. Without it, my friendships with these men would be much less enjoyable, owing to the great distance among us — might even, more likely, fade into nonexistence.

One day around four years ago I had an e-mail from a man who complimented me on something I had written; I cannot remember what it was. I answered, thanking him. He waited a decent interval, then sent me another e-mail, which engaged my attention with a penetrating question, which showed him to be a man with powers of intellectual insight.

Living in a small town in the South, he has had a hunger for the literary life that could not be met there or at the college in which he taught for thirty years. He has a wife whom he adores and a son in his twenties, but, now retired, he spends much time alone. He has no taste for travel. Perhaps a man of imagination doesn't need to travel: the poet Wallace Stevens, for example, never made it to Europe. What this man does is read, with intensity and care. He has a great fondness for poetry and has read the Anglo-American literature canon, from Chaucer to F. Scott Fitzgerald, in a thoughtful and impressive way. An amazon.com man, he also makes an effort to read good contemporary writing. He has excellent literary taste and judgment. While literature is the source, perhaps the deepest source, of pleasure in his life, it also distances him from the people around him. This is one of the negative, sad effects of culture that is seldom mentioned.

He also has a central sadness in his life: the death of one of his two sons, who died in a brutal way. I didn't find out about this loss until a good while after our e-mail correspondence had begun. He told me about it when in the grip of a lengthy dark phase in his life. Fitzgerald, who died before he qualified as middle-aged, once said that the natural state of a middle-aged man should be one of mild depression. What he meant was that, from the onset of middle age, death begins to hover uncomfortably closely, and one hasn't the freedom (which really means the time) to undo the mistaken decisions one has made, or to accomplish the dreams one had when young, or to turn to some new endeavor; life's essential finitude becomes all too real.

I hope this man will agree with me when I say that his reasonable middle-aged depression takes more radical dips than does mine, which is more steady-state. In any case, neither of us is fit to address the Rotary luncheon next Tuesday. This may be one of the things we find agreeable about each other. But I also think we share a point of view: we each have a pretty strong notion of how, in the larger scheme of things, insignificant we are.

He lives amid nature, I live amid human nature, and so we both see our share of red tooth and claw. We fancy ourselves realists, except that we both hope for some glimmer of wisdom before the lights go out—and I don't mean all over Europe or in the gardens of the West but in our own mild lives.

He has the diarist's impulse. He records the everyday incidents in his life: one of his large dogs kills a pig; he visits an insane cousin who believes he is God; a large snake crosses his path at a nearby pond; he runs into a former student while taking his wife to dinner at a barbecue restaurant. He will have read a poem, a line in which reminds him of a high school teacher who, like other such selfless people, has now, as the poet whom he quotes (Donald Justice) says, "stepped off to their doom."

He was a good high school athlete—played baseball and football—in a small town, where such prowess made one, briefly, a golden boy. My own athletic career was less golden—more like copper—but we each remember how heroic boys older than we once seemed to us. We were both in the peacetime army, and have that experience, too, in common. Each of us floated into an interest in literature without our knowing exactly how this happened when everything in our respective but very different backgrounds would seem to have militated against it.

He initiates most of our exchanges, which can number from one to four or five a day. Recently retired from teaching, he has more free time than I do. (If he had sent me four or five letters a day, I should no doubt long ago have cut loose of the relationship out of sheer fatigue.) Not all of his e-mails call for an answer. His e-mails tend to be longer than mine; my answers, I fear, sometimes border on the terse. Occasionally he will ask my advice: What is the best English edition of Proust? (I tell him the Terence Kilmartin edition.) Should he, being apolitical, subscribe to the *New York Review of Books*? (Yes, but only for the literary and historical stuff.) Sometimes he wishes to check his own reactions against mine: What do I think of a John Updike story in the current *New Yorker*? All this makes it sound as if I am the senior man in this friendship. In fact he will not infrequently mention some book or quote from a poem with the most useful consequences for me. He put me back onto rereading and reading about Samuel Johnson, a figure in his pantheon of writer heroes; John Keats, Emily Dickinson, Joseph Conrad, Henry James, Willa Cather, and Wallace Stevens are others in that pantheon. The street, in other words, has been far from one-way in this electronic friendship.

From his e-mails over the years, I know a good deal about his daily routine: his walks along a pond with his dogs, the name of his cat, his neighbors (both kindly and crazy), his boyhood friends, his daily workouts (he does an appallingly high number of sit-ups, even for an ex-jock), his heavyset mailwoman Peggy, his drink of choice (bourbon and Coke), his reading habits, his deliberately limited social life, his love for his wife, his sense of being impressed by the mysteries of life, and his confidence that they are not finally to be fathomed by we human beings before we depart the earth for certain oblivion. But this is knowledge accumulated over many months. A more typical e-mail will be a snapshot-like paragraph of a small incident:

> I took the dogs to the pond a bit earlier today. I have a man coming early this afternoon to do some work about the house; for one thing, to run a new electrical wire to the weight room. It was a splendid day for a walk, a quintessential autumn day, comfortably cool, the sky, devoid of clouds, full of bright light. Our walk was pretty much uneventful, until we got back to the truck itself. While I tried to load the dogs, they ran about my truck, both of their noses aquiver, both of them excited, intense and agitated, neither of them paying a bit of attention to my impatient adjurations. I thought that men are visual, but dogs interpret the world through their sense of smell. Wonders come though their noses; coherence is olfactory. With minor difficulty, I managed to get the dogs loaded. As I drove the hundred yards or so down the dirt lane to the main highway, I glanced over into the pecan grove beside the road and saw standing under a huge pecan tree a red fox. No doubt the fox is what my dogs smelled. Perhaps it had come by my truck. I had no doubts: this was a fox I saw, and when I saw the fox I realized with almost complete certitude that the animal I saw the other day was a coyote since it was considerably larger than the fox. How brazen, I thought, of the fox to stand in the open the way he was doing. I can't say for sure, of course, but the creature standing beneath the pecan tree looked imperturbable to me. His head seemed to follow me as I drove past. I got a good look at the fox, found it to be a handsome creature, winsome, graceful and nimble looking.

Often he will send me an interesting squib of poetry — from W. H. Auden or Wallace Stevens or Robert Frost — which will lead him to make an observation, to which I answer with my own. He seems to have no difficulty telling me what he thinks about life, nor do I hesitate to reply to his views.

This man, about the details of whose everyday existence I have come to know so much, is also someone I am fairly sure I shall never meet. He once sent me, via computer, a photograph of him and his wife. (He has some notion of what I look like from book jacket photographs.) I once telephoned him about some literary business I did with him and discovered he has a strong Carolinian accent, reminiscent of *The New Yorker*'s Joseph Mitchell. I felt he was a touch nervous when we spoke over the phone. His preferred medium is, apparently, the computer, specifically e-mail.

I'm not sure we need to meet. We might be disappointed. Our wives might not cotton to each other, or to one or the other of us. But, then, we're fine as we are, I think, and I suspect that he thinks so, too.

And yet I have come to consider this man, whom I have never seen but for whom I have great regard, among my good friends. Ours is a friendship of a kind undreamt of by Aristotle, Cicero, Montaigne, Saint Augustine, or anyone else alive before the late twentieth century. I owe this friendship to a technological advance. Despite what the Bible says, apparently there are new things under the sun.

# 16

❖

## *Friendship's New Rival*

"My FRIENDS MEAN everything to me," said the man sitting across from me in the Spanish restaurant, his face taking on a grave look that was at odds with his normally sly and ironic style. He was not yet forty and still a bachelor. As he said it, I thought that not many married men today would say something similar, with the same earnestness, though I could imagine a married woman saying it.

Marriage is one of life's great dividers. For one thing, it can divide — or should divide, given the responsibilities it brings — a person's life between extended adolescence and adulthood. (True, some married people remain children; in marrying they just bring their toys together under one roof.) For another, more obviously, it divides the married from the unmarried. And if the marriage turns out to be a genuinely close one, it can also divide a couple from the rest of the world. I have heard people complain that one of the problems of their upbringing was that their parents loved each other too much, so that they never felt that they, as children, could break into the tight circle of intimacy between them. The historian Edward Gibbon was such a person, and in his *Memoirs* he remarked that his parents were so wrapped up in each other that he felt he was never of more than peripheral interest to them.

More to the point, marriage divides friends, often the very closest of friends. Once one of them is married, two men who have been close friends are likely to find certain subjects no longer up for discussion: the comedy of chasing women is but one notable example. I first married at the age of twenty-three, and though I was not sorry to be married, I can recall feeling a slight but sad distance set in among my bachelor friends and me. An invisible electric fence had been put up, and they and I were now on different sides of it. We stayed in touch, continued to see one another with some regularity, but the terms of our friendships had fundamentally altered. I awaited these friends' own marriages — some, forty-odd years later, still haven't made it — so they could join me on my side of the invisible fence.

Marriage often entails a circling of the wagons. When children arrive, the circle is sometimes drawn closer, tighter. But the need for another distinction arises. There are of course good marriages and bad, but within even good marriages there are those in which husband and wife are best friends and those in which they are not, or at least not quite, or not at the same intensity, seamlessness of interest, and selfless devotion that the deepest friendships often have.

I have lived in both a bad and a good marriage, and the difference is that my second wife is easily my best friend in a way that my first wife and I, being very young, never contemplated being. If ever you wish to feel utterly friendless, my advice is to arrange to live a few years in a bad marriage. To live in a bad marriage is to be confronted daily with your poor judgment, to know disappointment, embarrassment, sadness, and shame, all more intimately and intensely than you ever expected.

To live in a good marriage, one in which husband and wife, along with being a legal entity, are also the best of friends, is to know friendship to the highest power — a power different yet perhaps higher than Aristotle, Cicero, and Montaigne imagined. Santayana, in *The Life of Reason*, writes: "The tie that in contemporary society most nearly resembles the ancient ideal of friendship is a well-assorted marriage. In spite of intellectual disparity and divergence in occupation, man and wife are bound together by a common dwelling, common friends, common affection for children, and, what is of great importance, common financial interests." Even more significant, as Santayana says elsewhere when defining a friend, it is with a husband or wife that one can be most human, or most oneself.

Marriage is obviously a legal arrangement, a form of partnership, but when the element of strong friendship is added it becomes something much more. And a friend in marriage is someone with whom you can, into the bargain, make love. (I earlier noted that friendship and sex do not mix; but in a good marriage they can and, with a bit of luck, will, with friendship over the years emerging as the much stronger element.) Toss children and, later, grandchildren into the relationship and marriage becomes a blood bond. Unlike the sanguinity at the heart of one's relationship with parents and brothers and sisters, however, marriage is freely chosen. To be in a marriage with a man or woman who becomes one's best friend — companion, confidant, lover, pal, all these things in one — is probably untoppable.

I knew a couple with nearly congruent intellectual and artistic interests, and I remember smiling when, years ago, the husband told me that he and his wife frequently stayed up till two or three in the morning, because once they got started on a subject, they couldn't bear to stop until they had drained it of all interest. And what did they talk about? The arc of John Dos Passos's career, whether James T. Farrell was a genuinely good writer, if Lionel Trilling was a more profound critic than Edmund Wilson. Granted, that may not be everyone's idea of a good time, may be more than most of us would want or could take, but it made this marriage an unending co-ed pajama party of a very sweet if sometimes exhausting kind.

Marriages in which husband and wife are best friends are also, by their nature, exclusive. They implicitly declare that any competition for being the best friend to either the husband or wife is closed, for the occupant of that post has long ago been declared, the position permanently filled, and the most anyone can hope for in the ranking of friendship is a distant second.

Where the complications in even superior marriages begin is in the friendships that couples in such marriages establish with other couples. Most of my parents' friendships were with other couples, though in my recollection none of them were all that close. My mother, whose gift for friendship, as I've noted, was much greater than my father's, was usually the pivotal person, the playmaker, in her and my father's meetings with other couples — that is, my mother and a female friend of hers would go out for dinner or a show with their husbands in tow. It was all pleasant enough, my guess is, but I don't believe anything magical happened, in the way it can when four people, all of whom enjoy one another's company immensely, are together.

My wife and I have known such magic, but with only a small number of couples over the thirty years of our marriage. A four-way reciprocity of good feeling and regard must be present for this to happen. Neither husbands nor wives must be along for the ride; not even one person can be outside the circle of affectionate feeling. No one person may be permitted to dominate the flow of talk. When this four-way friendship works, it is surpassingly charming, sweet, lovely, a fine game of doubles with four evenly matched players all of whom are dedicated not to winning but to keeping the ball in play.

My wife and I long ago discovered that the chief criterion for finding another couple congenial is that they, the other couple, must love each other. If they do not, if they just get along, if they have long ago merely come to terms with each other, it doesn't work. And if they dislike each other, then such a four-way friendship isn't anywhere in the realm of possibility.

Yet in the case of those couples my wife and I have most enjoyed being with in their capacity (as the philosophers would have it) *qua* couples, events have intervened to separate the four of us: death, divorce, and moving away have broken the magic circles. We know other couples with whom we think such magic might prevail, but inevitably they live in other cities, so our meetings as a foursome are too infrequent to be put to the full test of friendship.

A friend of mine who thought he had several splendid relationships with other couples learned, upon his wife's death, that he no longer had any interest in being with these couples.

They were welcoming enough to him, but without his wife on the scene such pleasure as he once knew among these friends had departed.

Divorce in some ways presents the most dramatic problem to these four-way friendships. If the divorce is a bitter one, you and your husband or wife are often left to choose sides, for the likelihood is great that the bitterness of one or the other member of the now divorced couple will not approve your seeing both of them, at least not on equal terms. Simply liking a divorced friend's new gentleman or lady friend might be viewed as disloyalty to the former husband or wife. But even when the divorce is amicable, complications set in. An obvious example is when one or the other of the former pair takes up with a man or woman who seems much less attractive than his or her former mate. When this happens, don't bother calling all the king's horsemen or all the king's men—the foursome is finished, the old magic never to be put back together again. Usually all that is left is the exercise of guarded tact and pretense.

Whether this speaks to my wife's and my high standards in friendship, or to our fragility both individually and as a couple, I leave it to readers to judge, but we have never chosen to travel for more than a few days with another couple. (Though we have, while traveling, met couples of whom we discovered ourselves fond.) Perhaps two weeks traveling with another couple in a foreign country would be the real test of couple friendship. We, though, have thus far decided not to attempt it, and my guess is that we shall probably depart the planet without doing so.

Marriage also puts in question the status of friends made before the marriage by either the husband or wife. In his essay "A Bachelor's Complaint of the Behavior of Married People," Charles Lamb remarked on the comic, though real, complications of being the friend to a man before and after his marriage. "Marriage by its best title is a monopoly," he writes, "and not of the least invidious sort." Before the marriage, in Lamb's case, was invariably better than after. A lifetime bachelor, Lamb was in a good position to know. (He never considered marriage for himself because he was guardian and devoted companion to his sister Mary, a gentle soul who suffered psychotic episodes, during one of which she stabbed her mother to death.) Lamb recounts the many ways wives have of chipping away at what one may have thought the granite of old friendships between men, and enumerates the many ways that a bachelor can be made to feel uncomfortable in a marital home. (Husbands can, of course, exert a similar and no less devastating talent in dealing with the old friends of their wives.) Lamb makes the point that his friendships with married men have been stronger with men he met after they had already been married than those with whom he had been friends before their marriages:

> But if the husband be a man with whom you have lived on a friendly footing before marriage, — if you did not come in on the wife's side, — if you did not sneak into the house in her train, but were an old friend in fast habits of intimacy before their courtship was so much as thought on, — look about you — your tenure is precarious — before a twelvemonth shall roll over your head, you shall find your old friend gradually grow cool and altered toward you, and at last seek opportunities of breaking with you. I have scarce a married friend of my acquaintance, upon whose firm faith I can rely, whose friendship did not commence *after the period of his marriage*.

I can testify to the high truth quotient of Charles Lamb's observation from both sides, married man and bachelor. The reasons why I retain some of my friendships dating back to high school are close to incomprehensible to my wife, who is not an imperceptive or intolerant person. Friends who seem to her without any interest in the things I have become passionately interested in, with whom I would not begin a friendship if I met them today, or thirty years ago, nonetheless remain my friends, if no longer always close ones. They do so because we have been through wars and amusing times together, and they retain qualities that I still value in them: a good heart, a strong sense of humor, or an outlook bred and developed in the solid philistinism of our old neighborhood which I continue to find of interest.

I can remember one night, not yet out of the army, still a

bachelor, meeting an old friend and his wife for dinner and being ferociously attacked by his wife for everything I said, most of which I thought was mild and uncontroversial. His wife, whom I had not met before, clearly loathed me at first sight. My friend chose not to speak during this verbal pummeling. (Their marriage, I later learned, was in trouble because of his drinking, and my guess is that she must have taken me for one of his drinking buddies.) Years later she gave a dinner to which she invited my wife and me, and she went out of her way to be kind to me. But my friendship with her husband never regained its old sure and delightful footing, and now that we are in late middle age, even though she is dead, I realize it never will.

Is the deep closeness of husband and wife a more traditionally American than European desideratum? Stories abound of more distant but still quite workable marriages among the European upper classes, in which freedom is built in, allowing for husbands and wives to take lovers. There are many jokes on the subject, such as that about the recently widowed Frenchman who has had a mistress he has seen every Saturday night for forty years and whose virtues he habitually extols. When a friend remarks to him that, now that his wife has died, he is free to marry his mistress, the man replies: "What? Marry my mistress? Impossible! What would I do with my Saturday nights?"

In America, far from reducing or delimiting a woman's friends, marriage can often increase and widen her range of friends. Many women now in their sixties and seventies fondly recall friends made at parks near their homes, where they took their children when the kids were very young, and there they met other young mothers with whom they had many interests in common. Some of these relationships, and other, newer ones, were—and continue to be—made through PTAs and various school organizations, children again providing the binding power here. A great number of these friendships stuck, growing stronger over the years.

You would think that Little League, junior hockey, soccer, and other sports do something similar for men, allowing them to meet fathers at the same stage of domestic and economic life as they. But even in this day of shared and co-parenting, of widespread joint custody and stay-at-home fathers, in most cases children remain the chief province of women, and those women who stay at home raising their children have more time than men to develop these friendships further.

Owing to the ever higher degree of attention that parents pay to their children — child-rearing, you will have noticed, is today a full-court-press affair, with everyone very nervous about it — the family may be emerging as one of the unspoken enemies of friendship outside marriage, a point I touched on earlier. A middle-class man of our time, a husband with children at home, figures to have a crowded life. Assume he works an eight-hour job — though if he is ambitious, ten or more hours is more likely to be the case — then add another two hours for getting to and from work. He is under greater pressure than at any point in history to spend more time with his children. He is under an obligation, too, to be a more attentive husband — an obligation greater than it once was, when the man, as sole breadwinner, was the figure in the household to whom attention had to be paid and around whom, when he was at home, most activities centered.

As like as not nowadays, this man's wife also works, and if he is not obtuse he will realize that he must share more than ever in household chores: shopping, caring for the kids, doing the laundry, perhaps much more. His weekends are unlikely to be as free as they once were. If he has a taste for sports, he probably will spend time in front of the television set or on the golf course or the tennis court; if he has a taste for books, he will try to slip off for a bit of reading. The one sure thing is that friends will have a lower priority than before he was married. Perhaps he will meet them every so often at a sports event, but he is more likely to do so on a social occasion with wives and possibly children present.

Because of the incursions of the family, institutions, both formal and informal, that were a regular part of masculine life fifty years ago currently seem to be diminishing, if not dying out. The weekly poker games, the bowling leagues, the adult fraternities (Knights of Columbus, Masons, et cetera), the boys' night out — one hears less and less of such purely male activities, at least among the middle class, where they seem to have lost their centrality. Men may now go to the gym, but the workout, for the purpose of retaining health to extend life, is much different from camaraderie, which is, or at least used to be, about useless fun that came under the heading of simply enjoying life. But now wife, children, family, and personal health come first.

The saddest dilemma is when two good things come into conflict. For it may well be that the family, certainly a good thing in itself, has become one of the greatest rivals of friendship, surely another good thing. Both have become more complicated than once they were. When they were, or at least seemed, less complicated, they weren't, or at least didn't appear to be, in conflict. There seemed time and room enough in most people's lives for both.

In a highly child-centered society, where above all attention must be paid to kids lest they grow up to be murderers — or, worse luck, do not get into Brown — friendship cannot compete. Friendship sometimes requires sacrifice and always requires outlays of time, but it goes without saying that none of this must be allowed to cut into time spent with one's family. Even when one no longer has children at home, the claims of friendship usually remain at best secondary. Can one be expected, for example, to lend ample sums of money to a friend when one's own grown children or young grandchildren may one day require financial help?

Today anyone who suggested that the claims of a friend ought to take precedence or to compete on an equal footing with those of a husband or wife or one's children would be thought monstrously mistaken. In any competition between friendship and family, friendship, bet on it, will lose every time.

In a good marriage there oughtn't to be any rivalry between husband and wife and the friends of each, but often there is. Sometimes a superior marriage will use up much of the social oxygen available to both parties. The more involved and in love with each other a married couple are, the less time they are likely to have for — or wish to spend with — friends, even dear friends. Jealousies can insinuate themselves. Why should my wife's — or husband's — friends occupy so much of the time, not to speak of affection, that by right belongs to me? Why is she always on the phone with her girlhood friends? Why would he want to go off for a weekend with his old college roommates? It can also work the other way around. "My true friends have always given me supreme proof of devotion," wrote Colette in her memoir *Break of Day;* "a spontaneous aversion for the man I loved."

Other complications for friendships follow upon marriage. One finally reconciles a good friend to one's husband or wife when — lo! — that friend up and marries someone whom both you and your wife dislike. Children can throw a heavy monkey wrench into friendships by being demanding, or inherently unattractive, or otherwise difficult. In "A Bachelor's Complaint," Charles Lamb remarks that for him "children have a real character and essential being of themselves; they are amiable or unamiable per se; I must love or hate them as I see cause for either in their qualities." Of course this was part of Lamb's problem. Even if the children are loathsome, if they are the children of friends they must be treated as lovable — for a guileless person not always an easy thing to bring off.

My parents were each other's best friend, though in a way that is likely to seem strange today. They were friends partly because, as I mentioned in an earlier chapter, my father was, outside his marriage, by choice pretty much friendless, and he required no network of friends. My mother's social gifts were more capacious; she was also, I came to think, much subtler in her judgments about people. But my mother loved my father without any hesitation that I could ever note, and I would be astonished if I were to discover that my father ever cheated on my mother.

Loyalty was at the center of my parents' marriage. As a clever child, I knew there was no way I could divide them to gain my own childish ends: theirs was a united and impregnable front. No one would think to speak ill of my father in my mother's presence. I have known a few occasions when her feelings were hurt on his behalf: once when they visited a family of cousins, the men went off to play golf, leaving my father, a nongolfer, behind. My father, so far as I knew, didn't seem to mind, yet my mother was furious and didn't speak to these cousins for years.

She could also play him for her own benevolent ends, suggesting he expend his natural generosity on her less well-off sisters and their children, on his and her own children, and on charities close to her heart. Her gentle nudging helped him to give way to his best instincts.

They were not an openly affectionate couple. I don't recall often seeing them kiss or embrace each other. When they argued, it was a brief flare-up, usually staged by my father, who felt that he was being pushed too far or that my mother was exceeding her authority by attempting to force decisions on him that he wasn't ready to make. The anger never lasted; I suspect they never took any bad feeling to bed with them.

Most extraordinary of all, they were amazingly, staggeringly reticent. My mother and father were married for fifty-seven years, before my mother died, of a slow cancer, at the age of eighty-two. One night, returning from visiting her in the hospital, where she was being treated for the liver cancer from which she eventually died, I asked my father what he knew about my mother's father, who had died when she was in her late adolescence and was a subject on which she had always been a good deal less than forthcoming. "Oh," my father said, "your mother's father committed suicide, but your mother doesn't know that I know."

My father then told me that he had found out about this from one of his sisters-in-law. But what I found astonishing was, first, that my mother had never mentioned this prime fact of her life to him, her best friend, through their long marriage, and, second, that he never told her that the fact was known to him. For fifty-seven years, neither felt any need to acknowledge to the other this momentous event in my mother's life. In our therapeutic age, this seems not merely astounding but close to nuts. They, however, lived comfortably enough with it. Had I asked my mother why she never told her husband about it, my guess is that she would have said that there was little point in dredging it all up, that talking about it wouldn't have made it any better.

After my mother died, my father, without his one dear friend, wandered in a desert of loneliness and unformulated anger at his loss. Then one day he betook himself down the hall of the high-rise building in which he lived and asked a woman he barely knew if he could take her to dinner. He was in his early eighties. She said she wasn't interested. He returned the next night to extend the invitation again, this time bringing flowers. They went out, then went out again, and yet again — and became a couple. She was six years younger than he. A widow, she was financially independent. They had in common a taste for foreign travel, for which she always insisted on paying her own way.

My father was mad about her. She took him with her to plays, movies, and concerts, things he did rarely with my mother. She was tougher on him than my mother had been, less patient with his large theories about the purposes of Mother Nature and the contradictoriness of humankind. My mother had let him do most of the talking; his new lady friend didn't mind cutting him off in mid-observation. From her he took interruptions, criticisms, and mild scoffing. With her shopping for his clothes, his style changed. When in his middle eighties he stopped driving, she chauffeured him. He was, my dear old father, clearly under new management.

For the last seven years of his life, they were constant companions. More than once my father told me how lucky he'd been to have had the affection of two such splendid women. He spent most nights at his lady friend's apartment. She prepared all his meals but his breakfasts, which he ate in his own apartment. He told me that he proposed marriage to her, but she wasn't interested, partly for the reason that if she married my father, the money due her as her husband's widow would be cut off. Besides, what difference might marriage make to their arrangement of almost constant companionship? My guess is that my father felt closer to this woman than he did to either of his two sons.

And then, at ninety, his body began to close down on him. He was diagnosed as having congestive heart failure; his heart was operating on progressively less oxygen, leaving him weaker and weaker. He was in a condition of dependency, which he hated. She stood by him, but at one point, when he began to wake seven and eight times a night to use the bathroom, out of restlessness, perhaps not getting sufficient oxygen while asleep, she said that she would like to speak with me. She told me that my father would have to return to sleeping in his own apartment, though she realized it would break his heart to do so. She was not planning to desert him, I was to understand. But she volunteered one morning a week at a nearby hospital; she also did volunteer work for her synagogue. She required her sleep. My father now needed someone on the premises full-time — he needed (sad word to apply to a paid stranger) a caregiver. His friend would continue to see him every day. She would eat most of her meals with him. But she had to go on with her own life. She was sorry, but she could not see any way around this. She hoped I would understand. And I did.

She was in every way well within her rights. My father, though saddened, understood, too. The only point I would make here is that similar behavior on the part of a wife or husband would have been intolerable. And therein lies one of the significant differences between a wife or husband and a friend: the latter does not, as the English say, have to see you out, has not signed on for the duration; before death the friend may, if the fancy takes him or her, depart. The nature of the two relationships, married partner and even dearest of dear friends, is fundamentally different, and there can be no doubt which, because more binding, is the stronger.

# 17

❖

## *Broken Friendships*

L IFE HAS NO PLEASURE higher or nobler than that of friendship," wrote Samuel Johnson in one of his *Idler* essays. "It is painful to consider that this sublime enjoyment may be impaired or destroyed by innumerable causes, and that there is no human possession of which the duration is less certain." Too true, I fear. So true, in fact, that it explains why the subject of broken friendships makes for the longest chapter in this book.

The best broken friendships are those that go unannounced and die on their own of inanition. The break itself entails no dramatic or sad scene, no inflamed emotion or smoldering anger, no climacteric whatsoever. These are friendships that, by unacknowledged agreement of both parties, are quietly allowed to lapse, no comment on either side. Whatever pleasure or promise one formerly felt in them somehow or other has gone, and past good feeling has, for various reasons, been allowed to leach away. All that is left is a grudging sense of duty, going through the motions, playing at charades of affinity that aren't any longer there. The hell with it, one or both parties to the friendship conclude, let it go.

Sometimes random events will make possible such breaks. One or the other of the friends moves away, or leaves the job that was the scene of regular meetings, or someone marries or divorces, which takes him or her out of the circle of exclusively married or exclusively single friends. But the vague dissatisfaction with the friendship is usually felt on both sides, so there is no truly injured party, no heavy freight of resentment hanging on afterward. "We had a lot of fun when we worked together at Allstate. I don't know what happened to him after he left the company. Nice guy, though."

Some friendships break down because time has altered old friends, given them different interests, values, points of view. However inevitable such ruptures are, there is nonetheless something sad about them. One friend may feel himself having become too large for the friendship, and may enjoy some (smug) self-congratulation that he has "grown" (always, I say, distrust botanical metaphors) so much more than his old friend. Meanwhile, the old friend is likely to feel confused or betrayed, probably thinking his friend more than a bit of a snob.

Sometimes, too, only one person works at the friendship, which can cause the other person eventually to drop away in discouragement. Truman Capote wrote accusingly to the critic Newton Arvin, who was once his lover and whom he wished to retain as his friend: "There are certain people with whom one can be the closest and most loving of friends — and yet they can quite quickly drop out of one's life simply because they belong to some odd psychological type. A type that only writes when he is written to, that only telephones when he is telephoned. That is — if one does not write him or telephone him one will never hear from him again. I have known several people like that, and this peculiarity of theirs, this strange eye-for-an-eye mentality, has always fascinated me." I first read that with a twinge, for alas I tend to be such a person. When there are two such friends, each awaiting word from the other, their friendship can only, in much less than the fullness of time, dissolve into indifference before going into full bankruptcy.

Some friendships break down owing to too thin a layer of common interest between the friends. In my thirties I met a man who was the athletic director at a gym to which another friend occasionally took me. This man was a few years older than I. When we met, I mentioned that I recalled that he had been an all-state football player when we were both in high school. "May I hug you for remembering?" he said, half jokingly. He was still a fine athlete. He also happened to be a wine expert, and one without the least trace of pretension. We would meet every so often for lunch. He offered to teach me about wine, though I decided not to take him up on the offer, feeling there was too much material of too little significance for me to attempt to memorize and master. Once we went out as a foursome with our wives. A few years later, he was undergoing a divorce, and he asked my help in writing letters to his soon-to-be ex-wife, which I was pleased to do. He seemed to be a man without malice: handsome, physically talented, with a swell smile, optimistic about life, a good guy in every way.

I had nothing but fondness for him, and yet in time we drifted apart. He left the athletic club and worked at a locally famous wine shop. Every so often someone told me that he saw him there. I suspect he is remarried; I hope he got it right the second time. If I were to run into him today, it would be, more than fine, damned pleasant. I hope he feels much the same toward me as I do toward him. Yet neither of us picks up the phone to call the other. Perhaps we had taken our friendship as far as good feeling could take it. Something else had to kick in to make it more than it was. Strange, but this is the way things often work.

A friend of mine, a woman who is a retired physician, not long ago told me that she is glad she no longer lives in New Orleans, so she doesn't have to spend so much time with the girls who went to school with her there. After she said this, she quickly added, "And I don't mean this in any self-congratulatory way, as if I have become more sophisticated or smarter than they." Why would she feel the way she does? Possibly because she felt freer with fewer old connections to worry about, possibly because she wanted to widen her perspective in a way that life among old school friends would not have permitted. Many, I think, will understand her motives without having to have them explained. A lot of us wouldn't mind shedding a few old friendships that have grown tedious, burdensome, even a little sad.

Breaks in friendship do become uncomfortable when someone feels betrayed or the victim of injustice as a result of the

break. Or when one person feels that the other is not near fulfilling his end of the unspoken contract that is essential to all
friendships: the sense of rough equivalence isn't there. Sometimes a single act can snap a friendship: failure to repay a debt,
word getting back of something unkind said behind one's back,
strong disagreement about something thought to be a matter of
profoundest principle, a failure to come through during a crisis.
Not uncommonly, the effects of such acts are known only to one
of the two friends. But one is enough; as the French philosopher Alain remarked, the full force of the slap in the face is felt
only by the person receiving it.

No surprise here, but there is a slew of books about how
to recover from the breakup of friendships. Self-esteem (self-ep-
stein, as I prefer to think of it) is often central to the arguments
made in them, and there are lots of "unresolved issues." Much
labeling goes on: "toxic" and "negative" relationships are emphasized, and lists of potentially disastrous friends are offered
(the Promise Breaker, the Controller, the Interloper, the Taker,
and so on). The usual made-up anecdotes about not quite be-
lievable people are provided. In the end, one is told not to let
the loss of friendships get one down, but instead pull up one's
socks, or hire a therapist to help pull them up for you, and get
back in the game. The level of human complexity on display in
such works is about that of a Barbra Streisand song ("People
who need people . . ."), which probably ought to be playing in
the background when reading them.

No general rules exist covering broken friendships. Some
people fall into the same kinds of misbegotten friendships over
and over—just as others fall into hopelessly misbegotten ro-
mances—and need to examine why such a wretched pattern of
relationships has arisen in their lives. Others have an insufficiently subtle sense of themselves and of the world, and are
likely to end up with sadly broken friendships even if they con-
sult a psychotherapist before agreeing to shake hands with a
new person.

Some people have no real gift for friendship, and look to ostensible friends only to be let down by them and hence for their
value as future enemies. "He was inordinately vain and cantan-

kerous," wrote Max Beerbohm about the painter James Whistler. "Enemies, as he had wittily implied, were a necessity to his nature; and he seems to have valued friendship (a thing never really valuable in itself to a really vain man) as just the needful foundation for future enmity. Quarrelling and picking quarrels, he went his way through life blithely."

Beerbohm also discovered a kind of friendship made to be broken that he called *sympat,* a word he took from a Brazilian he met abroad who, after a few meetings, said to him, "Never, my friend, did I yet meet one to whom I had such a *sympat* as you!" In an essay using that charming neologism for its title, Beerbohm calls relationships made while traveling or on holiday *sympats.* He recalls the initial pleasure one feels when, in unfamiliar surroundings, one finds people with whom one has things in common, and consequently senses a more immediate closeness than one might feel with the same person at home. "*Sympat,*" Beerbohm writes, "is but the prelude to *antipat.*" Not, he claims, that one should avoid such friendships when away from home; the trick is to avoid meeting these people back home at all. The moral seems to be that friendship, like love, has its illusions when encountered abroad.

With Beerbohm's notion of the *sympat* in mind, I recall a time when I might have played a role resembling that of the dreary *antipat.* It had to do with the novelist Ralph Ellison, who had written an essay for a magazine I then edited. When I wrote to thank him for the essay, which was both beautiful and wise, he wrote back to invite me to lunch when next I was in New York.

I took Ellison up on his offer, and we met one wintry day at the Century Club for no less than four hours. Everything about our meeting seemed magical. Our flow of talk was unbroken: gossip, friends we had in common, the present state of writing, jokes, much laughter, and great good feeling on both sides. I had walked into the Century Club while it was light and walked out into the dark; the experience was like that of attending a brilliant, entirely pleasing afternoon movie. I had met a man I had long admired and found him not in the least disappointing. I felt I had made a new friend.

When I returned to Chicago, I wrote Ellison a note of thanks for the lunch and the splendid afternoon. I added that I hoped he would let me know if he planned to be in Chicago, so I could stand him to a similar lunch. No answer arrived to this note. A month or so later I wrote again, this time inviting him to write another essay for my magazine. No answer. A few months later, I wrote to tell him some bit of news that I thought might interest him. Again nothing. Ellison and I never had another communication of any kind.

Not long after he died, I had a letter from a reader the last paragraph of which asked if I knew Ralph Ellison. He and his wife, this man reported, were on a cruise and met Ralph and Mrs. Ellison, with whom they hit it off (he thought) beautifully. When they returned home, he wrote to Ellison not once but several times, but no reply ever arrived. Did I, he wondered, have any explanation for this strange behavior?

I now think the explanation may be in Max Beerbohm's notion of the *sympat.* Ralph Ellison was a naturally gregarious man. He was a man whom many people, I among them, would have been pleased to think of as a friend. He was also a man who in 1954 had published a fine novel, *Invisible Man,* and hadn't written another during the decades since—a man, in other words, haunted by work undone. He didn't need more friends filling up his days with correspondence, lunches, and the other time-consuming niceties following from his natural sociability. No *sympats* for Ralph, evidently; he eliminated them before they had a chance to turn *antipat.* Because he was so charming a man, I had personal reasons to regret this, but I now think I understand it.

"No true hatred is possible except toward those one has loved," wrote Paul Valéry in his *Notebooks.* I don't know what occasioned this dark remark, which I quoted earlier. Valéry may have intended it to apply to lovers, but it also has its application to parties to a broken friendship. The broken friendships that turn to hatred most readily are those in which one had the most feeling invested before the break.

*Embers,* by the Hungarian writer Sándor Márai, is a fine novel for which Valéry's aphorism might serve as an epigraph.

Set in the late Austro-Hungarian Empire, it is about two boys who befriend each other at an early age, go through school, then officer training school, and their early manhood together. Their steadily deepening friendship, despite the discrepancies in the wealth of their respective families, is beautifully built up by the author; it is something each had planned to last a lifetime, something dear, almost sacred, demanding unconditional honor and loyalty.

A break of many decades follows, during which one of them goes off to work in the colonies. The setting for the novel is the home of the wealthier of the two friends, now a widower, who has invited his old friend for dinner at his estate. Both men are now perhaps in their seventies.

At this dinner, the host carefully explains that he has discovered that this dear (or so he always believed) friend has had a love affair with his wife. His learning of the affair chilled, and in effect killed, his marriage, for although he and his wife remained married, they subsequently lived separately on his large estate, avoiding seeing each other after the betrayal was revealed. Now that she is dead, her husband feels he must confront his old friend with what he knows.

What he learns is that his friend and his wife were united by a love of music, which both played and were enraptured by, and which was largely closed off to him. They met on a ground — the artistic — to which he was in effect denied entry. Still, the betrayal was fundamental. It went so far that this friend contemplated killing him when he was out hunting, so he could live with his wife. He gains no real pleasure in confronting his old friend with all this; and the friend, far from seeming to squirm at being caught out, doesn't apologize — in fact he barely responds. Fate, not willed human action, the novel suggests, seems to have pulled the strings here. But at least now the books are cleared. In the cliché of our day, there is closure, and of a kind that is highly satisfying.

The reason "closure" is a cliché is that it is used too often, too imprecisely, and doesn't in any case reflect reality. In reality, such closure in broken friendships, and much else in life, is rarely achieved; only death brings closure, and then not always for those still living. The causes of most broken friendships are not so clear and clean as one finds them in even the best literature. In life closure turns out to be no easier to achieve than true repression.

I have searched my past and cannot think of a wrecked friendship that broke my heart—hurt feelings, yes—but I can think of one broken friendship the aftermath of which pestered me for an unhealthily long spell. That friendship was with someone with whom I had gone to high school and then to college, where for a year we had been roommates. In the stadium seating plan of my friendships, he held a box seat, very close to the field. We had ended up working at the same university, in the same English department, he as a senior professor, I as a sort of permanent visiting writer. This was during a time when English department studies were shifting dramatically, from straightforward examination of literary works for their most persuasive meanings to more politicized, sociosexual interpretations.

The details are too elaborate (and boring) to go into here, but an incident involving a highly radicalized teacher, who claimed not to believe in free speech (when it went against her views), divided many people in the English department. I could not fathom how anyone teaching in a university could be against free speech, and told my friend that I thought most people sided with the professor out of fear of seeming against the radicalism then still rampant in universities, which was in reality a variety of deepest conformism. Cowardice, I said, was the only explanation for such behavior. He then told me—what I had already known—that he was on the radical professor's side. Did I think him a coward? "I'm sorry to say I do," I said, realizing as I said it that I should have played for time here, searched for a euphemism, found some way not to call him a coward. But in the passion of the moment, I didn't. The words were out of my mouth and the friendship was over. The incident took place nearly twenty years ago. Safe—and sorry—to say that the friendship has not been, and likely never will be, renewed.

For weeks afterward, I found myself, at odd moments (before drifting off to sleep, in the shower, watching a baseball game), thinking angrily about what I took be my now ex-friend's spine-lessness. I felt confident (as, alas, I still do) about being right in our argument, but I also felt righteous, an emotion always to be distrusted. What were once ignorable flaws in my former friend now seemed more genuine expressions of what I took to be his general obtuseness. I mentally replayed such evidence as I could dredge up of his bad character, analyzed it, and attacked it over and over. Enough already, I would say to myself, put off by what seemed a pettiness in my need to rip the former friend apart, at least in my mind. It took me months to get clear of all the bitterness. Like the man said: "No true hatred is possible except toward those one has loved."

It saddened me, too, to think that politics was the cause of the dissolution of this once good friendship, since, though I have a politics, I prefer to think mine a personality far from dominated by politics. Disagreement over politics is probably among the leading causes of the breakup of friendships, at least among supposedly educated people for whom political opinion looms importantly. Differences over religion are not so great in strengthening friendships, either, but political disputes seem to ignite ugly emotions, to get things to the yelling stage, more quickly than anything else. In the eighteenth-century clubs and coffeehouses, politics was, quite sensibly, prohibited as a subject for discussion.

*Ex-Friends* is the title of a memoir by Norman Podhoretz about his broken friendships with various New York intellectuals, among them Lionel and Diana Trilling, Hannah Arendt, Norman Mailer, and Lillian Hellman, all once eminences in the intellectual life of the country. In each case, politics was at the heart of the disruption and eventual dissolution of the friend-ship, and Podhoretz, in what seems to me an attractively fair fashion — fairer, I think, than I should have been capable of doing — sets out in a clear and detailed way how each friend-ship fell apart.

I have known Norman Podhoretz and have written for *Com-*

*mentary,* a magazine he edited, for about forty years. We are good friends, though not close friends; we have never spent all that much time alone together in a way that would make a closer friendship possible. I like Norman and admire him, too, for he has taken positions based on his beliefs that have cost him and his family much unjustified contumely, and at times, I have no doubt, true anguish; at a minimum they cost him a secure place in what, snobbishly considered, was once a central place in the establishment version of American intellectual life.

Yet Norman is a polemicist, to the bone and beyond, and a polemicist is a professional arguer. (*Polemos,* in Greek, I am told, means war.) His has been a life lived in and through argument. Very near the pure type of the intellectual, he thrives on it. He is naturally contentious; he cannot avoid taking positions, cannot say other than what he thinks; candor is in his nature. He has more charm than diplomacy. He is a person who, if you happen to disagree with him, does not make it easy to like him, though he has commanded great loyalty among his friends in a way that speaks to a true gift for friendship.

Norman Podhoretz's problem is that he knows only one way to take ideas — and that is dead seriously. As he says in the introductory chapter of *Ex-Friends,* friends can disagree about a lot, "but only provided the things they disagree about are not all that important to them." He is far from alone in this; he is, in fact, in interesting company. In 1914, with World War I about to begin, Ludwig Wittgenstein wrote to Bertrand Russell: "I can see perfectly well that your value judgments are just as good as mine and deep-seated in you as mine in me, and I have no right to catechize you. But . . . for that very reason there cannot be any real relation of friendship between us."

When Norman Podhoretz turned away from his rather standard radical-left politics of the late 1950s and early 1960s, he came to believe what we all now know to be patently true: that the Communism then prevalent was a force for suffering and grief in the world and was worth fighting against; that socialism was an idea whose time had long passed and probably wasn't such a hot idea in the first place; that America was on balance a good place in which one was fortunate to find oneself living;

that sexual and identity politics traduced clear thinking. When he argued in print about these things, the house came down on him — also the landscape and a few clouds. He was looked upon by his former friends, he writes, "as a dangerous heretic, which," he adds, "I certainly was from their point of view, and I considered them a threat to everything I hold dear, which *they* certainly were — and still are." Those friends who did not think him stupidly or evilly wrong more charitably, one supposes, considered him insane. "No wonder, then," he writes, "that there is hardly a one of my old friends left among the living with whom I am today so much as on speaking terms, except to exchange the most minor civilities if we happen unavoidably to meet (and often not even that)."

Here is the question *Ex-Friends* raises in high relief: For what ideas would one be willing to give up one's friends? Most of us, I suspect, would say that there are no ideas, which are after all abstract things, worth a single friend, who is after all a flesh-and-blood person. Perhaps only intellectuals can break friendships over ideas, never for a moment to deny that ideas do have consequences in the world: Communism began as an idea and ended up causing death and misery to scores of millions of people for nearly a century. Recall that Cicero defined friendship "as nothing other than agreement over all things divine and human along with good will and affection." That is a lot to ask, but general agreement on major matters is still a great lubricant for a friction-free friendship.

As I said earlier, for me a person's point of view is more important than his or her opinions, though the line between the two, true enough, is not always easily drawn. Can a Jew, for a provocative example, continue a friendship with someone who approves of Palestinian terrorism? Can an African American ever overlook obvious racism in a person he calls friend?

Jean-Paul Sartre and Albert Camus broke up a friendship over Camus's book *The Myth of Sisyphus,* which argued that utopians are frequently the world's most dangerous people. Sartre, who, in the name of a far-off utopianism, found he could live comfortably with Stalin, felt this going altogether too far, and wrote Camus out of his circle of influence. (Today Camus's reputation for integrity and honor generally is much higher than Sartre's.)

Sigmund Freud broke with just about everyone in what was once called the Freudian circle: Carl Jung, Wilhelm Fliess, the entire group. Dominance of ideas was at stake, and Freud, as the leader of a powerful new movement, could not bear much deviation from his own central ideas, even from colleagues who were also friends. When one's subject is the understanding of human nature, as it was in modern psychoanalysis, a straight party line was unlikely to prevail, and the breakup of friendships, even those based on discipleship, was predictable.

George Orwell, who took ideas seriously enough for most tastes, wrote a letter to Stephen Spender touching on this point. The letter was written just after Orwell met Spender for the first time. In it Orwell writes that, until now, he always thought of Spender as the kind of person he despised: a Communist fellow traveler, an effete poet, a weak type all around. (Orwell was accurate in all this.) But, Orwell writes, having met Spender, he found him in person rather agreeable and therefore could never again attack him with the clean brutality that he formerly enjoyed in writing about him. Probably it is a mistake, Orwell concludes, to attend parties where he might meet other enemies, find himself liking them, and be unable further to attack them with a clear conscience.

How many friendships break down over conflicts in opinion and ideas cannot be known. My guess is that many more friendships fall apart through what are taken to be insults (many of them unintended), and wounds resulting from pride, ingratitude, feelings of abandonment, and misunderstandings. Pascal writes that "if everyone knew what one said of the other there would not be four friends in the world." The number four seems a bit high.

Many other friendships break down because one friend cannot take the other for what he is and feels he must try to reshape him into what he would prefer him to be. I once angered a good friend whom, when he was out of work, I tried too hard to push into taking on small writing jobs. He was a man who could write but didn't really want to write, and I of course should have known that without the desire behind it, writing is a torture. Unemployment had not put him in the best of moods in any case, and he told me to leave him the hell alone. We didn't speak for a few years afterward, and I missed him sorely.

The most vivid instance of trying to reshape a friend that I know was the effort on the part of my dear friend Edward Shils to reshape the character of his then friend Saul Bellow, a friendship I touched on earlier. The two men enjoyed a rough parity of prestige, Shils as an international scholar and Bellow as a literary artist, though Edward was four or so years older and the much stronger personality. He appreciated Bellow's talent but wanted him to be somehow grander, more dignified in his personal life than it was in him to be. He wanted Bellow to be Thomas Mann with Jewish jokiness added. Not an easy thing to be, granted, but had Bellow been able to bring it off, the result would have been immensely impressive.

Although Saul was already world famous and in his fifties, Edward did not see that as any reason not to attempt to reform him. Edward was a true teacher; he could not help setting people straight. Saul took a fair number of sermonettes from him, on what Edward considered the shabbiness of his conduct, without (expressed) resentment. Samuel Johnson, an unreformable handful of a human being himself, instructs that we must accept our friends as they are — by which he meant with all their tics and weaknesses and difficulties. "Take friends such as we can find them," he wrote, "not as we would make them." It's sound advice that Edward, in his reforming zeal, could not bring himself to accept.

I first came to know the two men on the eve of the breakup of their friendship. Saul Bellow had introduced me to Edward Shils. We were all unmarried at the time. Edward had brought Saul to the Committee on Social Thought at the University of Chicago. Some say that he converted him politically, making Bellow, a former Trotskyite, less sympathetic than he might otherwise have been to the student revolutionaries of the late 1960s. Edward's annotations on Bellow's *Mr. Sammler's Planet* are said to have been extensive, changing the book in important ways, and anyone who knew both men can feel his influence on that novel. The friendship must at one time have been very close and precious to both men.

When I came to know them, however, fissures, cracks, and lots of fallen plaster were already in evidence. Each would put down the other to me—brilliantly, I must say—sometimes in back-to-back phone conversations. When I told Saul that I had gone to dinner the previous night with Edward, he asked me if "Edward still has a leather palate" (behind the insult was Edward's reputation as a gourmand who was also a first-class cook). Edward called a few minutes later, and, after I had told him that I had spoken earlier with Saul, he said, "I was thinking that if our friend Saul were permitted to spend two hours in a tête-à-tête with the Queen of England, he would come away to make two observations: first, that she has no understanding of the condition of the artist in modern society, and second, that she is an anti-Semite." Edward never resisted a chance to put Bellow down. He began referring to Bellow, who had aged badly, as "the old gentleman," and I'm sure Saul had many equally debasing things to say about Edward, though I was no longer in touch with him to hear them.

Saul felt that Edward did not respect him sufficiently; Edward felt that Saul failed to heed his advice and continued to act badly. ("He is trying to make the Committee on Social Thought a retirement home for his old girlfriends by getting them jobs there," he once told me, "and I'll be damned if I'll let him turn the place into his personal bordello.") The two men pulled further and further apart as they continued to trade unpleasantries. As Edward lay dying, Saul asked if he might come to bid him a final farewell. Edward said he preferred that Saul not do so, eschewing sentimental farewells. After Edward had died, Saul, whose primary weapon of attack had always been his novels, put him in *Ravelstein,* where he is described by the title character as smelling musty and probably a homosexual, neither of which was remotely true. But this, again, is the kind of vicious stuff possible only among enemies who once loved each other.

Friendship sometimes resembles love in being subject to

jealousy. I should have liked to remain friends with both Edward Shils and Saul Bellow, but such was their rising enmity, I had to choose between them. I chose Edward—not abruptly but slowly, over a year or so—because he seemed more generous, more in need of a friend, and, lest I paint myself as blithely altruistic, because I took greater pleasure in his company and sensed that he was much the larger-hearted man. I don't for a moment think that Saul Bellow was jealous of my friendship with Edward Shils; I was never more than a secondary figure to him, however genially we got on.

But it is not uncommon for two close friends to resent a third party. Or, sometimes, for that third party to decide he or she resents the original closeness of the two friends. The novelist Paul Theroux blames the breakup of his once close friendship with the writer V. S. Naipaul on the latter's marriage to a woman he describes as an aggressive and interfering Pakistani journalist. Theroux's *Sir Vidia's Shadow* is his risibly vitriolic attempt to put Naipaul down by mocking his pretensions and highlighting his cold-bloodedness—at book length. "Friends provoked," notes the seventeenth-century writer Baltasar Gracián, "become the bitterest of enemies."

No friend has broken with me in recent years, though I have known a few people who, I have to assume, did not long for my company when I have offered it. A couple I have invited three or four times to join my wife and me for dinner have not acted on the invitation; I've now stopped asking. I do not think they despise me, but merely that they get on nicely without us. I have another friend, from college days, whom I see perhaps once every ten years, our meetings always ending with my remarking that we mustn't let so much time pass before our next meeting. He, however, seems content to let the time pass. Most strangely of all, I have a friend, also from college days, whom I hadn't seen for thirty years, then began seeing again with some frequency for four years or so, and now no longer see again. Apparently our friendship is on a four-years-on, thirty-years-off cycle, and clearly we do not have sufficient time left for another cycle. Did I offend him somehow? Or perhaps I unconsciously irked his wife. Might it be that I am not the charming fellow I believe I am? Good God, surely not.

I have broken off a few friendships myself, not all of them justly. A former student, who was never anything other than kind and respectful to me, and who went off to become a teacher himself, sent me a copy of a book he had written about the history of the teaching of creative writing in the universities. In it I am acknowledged in the same sentence with another teacher whose thinking I have always found unattractively dry and hopelessly obtuse. I dashed off a letter to my former student, telling him that having my name joined with this man's drained any pleasure his acknowledgment might have given me, and that, moreover, he couldn't possibly have been influenced by the two of us, else he would have to be schizophrenic.

I'm sorry I composed and sent that letter; I don't even have the excuse of the rapidity of e-mail composition to blame for it. I must have been in a foul mood the day I wrote it. I would have done better to have smiled and let it all pass. Some years later, when I wrote a memoir about my teaching days, this now no-longer-young man wrote a letter to the editor of the magazine in which it appeared to say how good a teacher he thought I was. I wrote to him to thank him for the letter and to apologize for my earlier offensive letter to him. But he never answered, which means that I needlessly, and perhaps permanently, hurt a friend.

Another friend sent me a book he was writing on Ernest Hemingway. He was a writer very much attuned to Freudianizing his subjects. Hemingway is of course choice meat for a biographer with such a tendency, for there is scarcely anything one can't do in the interpretative line with his super-masculine bravado. But my friend, I thought, was really pushing it; and in a response to one of the chapters he sent me, I wrote that he might be unaware of it but he seemed to be on the path to discovering that Hemingway was a repressed lesbian. He didn't find the comment amusing. His response to it, in fact, was to write to my wife, suggesting that I was in need of therapy. That snapped it.

A friend of his subsequently told me that he, my friend, suffered great intellectual insecurity while at work on his books, and would lash out when he suspected the least criticism. Mine was rather more than the least criticism. We didn't communicate again for fifteen years. Then, for reasons I cannot recall, he began writing me brief, friendly notes, which I always answered but in a deliberately distant manner. I had heard that he had been ill. I asked if we could meet for a drink when next I was in Washington, D.C., where he lived. When I met him, I was startled by how his illness had ravaged him. We easily slipped back into our old friendship; we had both reached the grandfather stage of existence; we still had a great deal to talk about. I instantly recalled why I had so much liked him.

Not long after this, I learned that he had cancer, from which he was likely to die. I bought an airline ticket to visit him at home, but at the last moment he had decided to check into Sloan-Kettering Cancer Center in New York for further treatment. He never came out. When I think about him today, I do not feel guilt so much as a sense of the lost good times we might have had together. All the laughter and good talk lost because of that stupid break in our friendship.

While not long ago reading Alice Munro's short story "Chance," I was struck by the following passage, pertaining to the story's heroine: "But she had also had the experience, for much of her life, of being surrounded by people who wanted to drain away her attention and her time and her soul. And usually she let them." I could, as they say, identify. A few times in recent years I have agreed to meet for coffee or lunch someone who, claiming to be eager to meet me after reading something or other that I have written, ended up by doing not half—which would be fair enough—but 80 percent of the talking, most of it about his or her own career. When this happens I make a mental note not to meet with that man or woman again, consider it an hour or so wasted, to be tossed into that garbage pile in the corner of every life that goes by the name of useless experience.

Sometimes relationships with which one is never too comfortable are allowed to run well past what should have been their reasonable limits and been quietly put to death. Thomas McGuane has a story on the subject called "Old Friends," about two men who meet in college, stay in touch over the years, and "become lifelong friends without ever quite getting past the fact that their discomfort with each other occasionally boiled over into active detestation." McGuane writes: "For decades, Briggs and Faucher had each been searching for an unforgivable trait in the other that would relieve him of this abhorrent, possibly lifelong burden. But, now that they had years of history and continuity to contend with, it had become harder and harder to imagine a liberating offense." Nothing for it sometimes but to forgo the search for that offense and make the break anyway.

Fifteen years ago I became trapped in a full-blown, one might almost say full-time, relationship of this kind that I found no way out of but cruelly to end it over the telephone. I knew going in that my partner in this relationship was neurotic, obsessional division, but I often don't mind neurotics, who sometimes have their own charm: Oscar Levant and George S. Kaufman come to mind. My friend, though, added a strong dose of solipsism to his neurosis, making for a strong brew.

In some ways, the basis of our friendship was our shared contempt for academics and intellectuals whom we thought naïve and artistically uncultivated. He could talk for great uninterrupted stretches about the awfulness of this or that writer or teacher or of the university scene. (I had written about these things, which relieved me of the burden of talking so much about them.) The problem, however, was in the word "uninterrupted." My friend was of the club of nonlisteners; he could have run for president of the club and won. I would attempt to break in, to add a point or give the conversation a slight turn, and he would mutter "Yeah, yeah," obviously not listening, and continue on his lecture or tirade.

Sometimes this got so bad that I would simply assert, "You're not listening," to which he would reply, "Yeah, yeah." Sometimes I would ask him to repeat what I had just said, which he usually couldn't do. He wanted to meet once a week, over coffee. I tried to get out of as many of these meetings as I could: I had already heard all his material, and I grew restive at having my own meager attempts at conversation so completely ignored. I used sometimes to say to my wife, "You meet him, please. It won't matter. All he really requires is a pair of ears into which to speak."

He could sometimes be amusing. He was often even interesting. He was in some ways generous. He was not by any interpretation a bad fellow, a man capable of mean acts. He just couldn't bear to listen. He couldn't do it, couldn't make himself do it. He had to keep talking; what he had was the affliction called logorrhea. He couldn't help it.

More and more often I made excuses for missing our regular sessions. Sometimes I would purposely not answer his calls (thank you, caller ID). But then he would leave messages saying he was worried about not hearing from me. Was I ill? Had something gone wrong in my family? He was, he said, concerned, and I don't doubt that he really was, or at least thought he was. He was—he is—a kindly man. The problem was that he couldn't stop talking, and after more than a decade I could no longer bear listening to him.

To reveal the extent of my social cowardice, it took me nearly two years to mount the courage to tell him that I wanted out, that he must find another set of ears, at least on Friday afternoons, the usual time of our meetings. I thought so much about how best to break with him that it interfered with my thinking about other things. Finally, one afternoon I called and told him that I wished him only well but that, since he couldn't seem to bring his nonlistening problem under control, I had decided to stop meeting with him. He felt, I sensed, that I was somehow ungrateful to him—or at least he used the word "ungrateful" in response to my awkward kiss-off. But in the end he manfully said, "Farewell, then, Joseph," and hung up the phone. I felt simultaneously terrible and hugely relieved.

Every broken friendship is a failure or defeat. It denotes poor judgment on one's part, or inflexibility, or insensitivity, or ungenerosity in one form or another. Yet are these sad relationships entirely without meaning? Nietzsche, who himself had a famous broken friendship with Wagner, whom he began by idolizing and ended by despising, has a strangely fortifying paragraph on the subject in *The Gay Science,* in which he tries to make lemonade out of the squishy lemon of broken friendships by suggesting that perhaps in "a tremendous but invisible stellar orbit such friendships might be renewed and better made." One would like to think this may be so, but the odds against it are only slightly higher than those on the return of vaudeville.

# 18

❖

## *Friendlessness*

"WE MAY CALL millionaires poor in respect to what they have not acquired or do not possess, and one may state that I too have grown poorer," wrote Libanius, the fourth-century (A.D.) Greek man of letters. "In fact one who does not say it has not, I think, adequately noted my circumstances, or how it would take a day to enumerate the friends of mine who have died."

At sixty-seven, I do not know precisely how many of my friends have died. Like Libanius, I've not set aside a full day to count. None of the early deaths in my wide circle of friendship were those of close friends, though most, it turns out, were extremely likable: a boy in high school who had kidney disease, a fraternity brother at the University of Illinois who went down in his twenties owing to a defective liver; each was a notably sweet character. Someone recently sent me a photograph of a club I belonged to in high school. Of twenty-odd boys in the photograph, four of the best-natured among us are now dead. A more actuarial mind than mine could no doubt work this out, but my guess is, should I live another ten years, which I am trying my best to do, at least a third, perhaps half, of my friends will have pegged out.

For a long while now it has been difficult to keep death, one's own and those of friends, out of mind. Henry James, in one of his letters, remarks that, upon reaching the age of fifty, he has discovered that someone he knows dies nearly every week. Given the increase in longevity since James's time, for me the age that this kicked in was sixty. Each week's obituaries in the *New York Times* presented me with the death of someone I knew or the friend or associate of someone I continue to know. Death, the Big D, "the distinguished thing" (as James is said to have called it on his own deathbed), closes in more insistently than one would prefer.

"But O the heavy change, now thou art gone," wrote Milton in "Lycidas" of his friend Edward King, drowned on the Irish seas. "Now thou art gone, and never must return." King died young, and one saw much opportunity for Lycidas-like sentiments in the 1980s and early 1990s, when the obituary columns were freshly filled with reports of the death of the young from AIDS.

"Loyalty in friendship is so rare and the dead so easily forgotten," wrote Pliny the Younger, "that we ought to set up our own monuments and anticipate all the duties of our heirs." Where in one's mental economy is room to be found for dead friends? In that increasingly blurry and discommodious instrument called memory, of course. When dead, we all naturally want to be remembered in the memories of our remaining friends. But how, and in what way?

Driving my granddaughter to school on a cold Thursday morning in late November, I noted two red paramedical trucks in front of the apartment building of a friend who had ALS, or Lou Gehrig's disease, one of the toughest of slow-death tortures. That afternoon I got a call from his son-in-law saying that he had died. His Filipina caregiver was bathing him and he just slipped away into death. He was seventy-seven. His ALS had advanced to the point where his speech was indecipherable, at least by me. The standard thing to say when a person in greatly debilitated or painful condition dies is that it was "a blessing." But a blessing for whom, exactly: the person who has died or his or her family and friends?

He was not a close friend, though without his ever getting gushy about it, he had revealed a few things about his life to me that one would normally tell only a close friend: some of his worries about his children, his disappointment over where the company he had run for many years was now headed under the control of new leadership, the differences in outlook between him and his wife, whom he nonetheless loved, and who had preceded him in death by two years. My guess is that he didn't have any truly close friends. He was an engineer by training and by outlook, which meant that he was exceedingly rational — to the point of claiming simply not to understand behavior that was stupid, self-destructive, crummy.

He was ten years older than I. When I was six or seven, he was the soda jerk at the drugstore — West's Pharmacy — at the corner of the block on which I lived, on Sheridan Road in Chicago. In those days he had a high pompadour and a bright winning smile. Several decades later — we had not met in be-tween-times — he called me one night to inform me, jokingly, that he intended to sue me because I had used his name for a crime syndicate figure in a short story I had written. I had done so by accident, for I had forgotten him and his name, but I offered to buy him lunch to make up for the use of his name.

When I met him, I recognized him straightaway: his hair was now white but still plentiful and still combed in a pompadour, his smile still commandingly charming, though it had taken on a touch of slyness. We talked about the old neighborhood, about the turns our lives had taken, about the state of the world, about the odd fact that we were once more neighbors. We agreed to meet again, and did, a few times a year, and then more often than that when he retired and had more free time.

Our conversations rambled from subject to subject: from baseball to politics to contemporary morality to the ways the world we were born in had changed for good and ill. He was very earnest, and had no aggressiveness to him that I could detect, which seemed unusual and therefore impressive for a man who had led a large company. When his wife died, a nimbus of loneliness hung over him; his sadness was palpable, though he never complained to me about it or, for that matter, about anything else.

I cannot remember the day he told me that he had been diagnosed with ALS, but soon after, he began to go down fairly quickly. We continued to meet for coffee, but he looked thinner, his left arm hung with unnatural looseness at his side, his speech became slightly slurred. Before long, he wasn't able to leave the house, and soon he required someone on the premises to help him bathe, get undressed, use the toilet, put on and remove an oxygen mask he was forced to wear, first at night and then throughout the day, too.

I visited him more frequently now that he was homebound, but still not all that often, perhaps once every three weeks. The downhill slope of the disease, in his case, was swift. At one point, he apologized to me for losing normal social self-control: "I just fart and belch away," he said. "Please forgive me." I told him that I didn't give a damn if he did so. Soon he had strength enough only to manipulate the remotes on his television and stereo system. He had a feeding tube inserted into his stomach. His throat was dry; he drooled; his head lolled to the side. Such was the muddiness of his speech that only his dear daughter and the woman who cared for him could make out what he was saying, and this usually after asking him to repeat himself two or three times.

I less and less looked forward to visiting him, even though I now never stayed more than an hour. I tried to time my visits to when baseball games were on, so that, with the television going, not much talk was required between us. I came only when I knew his daughter would be there, to serve as my interpreter. I brought him CDs—Jack Teagarden, Louis Armstrong—because he could still enjoy music. But I felt terrible, for his bad luck in having this wretched disease, for my own uselessness, and for the limits of friendship when another person has been kicked in the teeth by life. I was, in the clichéd phrase, "there for him," though I cannot see that it much mattered.

Not, I am sure, that he expected any more from me. He was probably pleased enough to see me, to know that I hadn't entirely forgotten about him. But what would he have thought about my reaction to his death? It's a blessing, I thought, in the approved manner. I felt gratitude in part for his escaping more physical torture but in just as great part for the relief in not having to continue my sad and hopeless visits to his apartment.

He is gone, dead, and I shall not again bump into him on the street. Each of us considered the other a friend; I think we respected and liked each other a lot; but neither thought of the other as a best friend or a particularly close friend. Yet, considered selfishly, his death diminishes me, depopulates my life, is a brick removed from the edifice of my past.

The metaphor of an edifice—from a cozy bungalow to a high-rise—for a lifetime's worth of friendships and acquaintances has a certain appeal. It helps to understand friendship as something one builds up and one stands by and watches being dismantled, by illness, alienation, and death, brick by brick—that is, if one is lucky enough to be reasonably long-lived and not oneself one of the early removed bricks. "We must either outlive our friends you know," remarked Samuel Johnson, "or our friends must outlive us; and I see no man who would hesitate about the choice."

And yet there is a pleasure in recalling dead friends, especially if they had been winning. Whenever I see a man in a heavy leather coat, I think of my friend Martin, who died in his middle forties and who had a thick, fur-collared leather coat that looked like just the thing for leading a Wehrmacht division at the Russian front during World War II. I always joked with him about that coat, and in postscripts to the letters we sent each other after he moved to London, I invariably inquired about the coat's well-being. Martin died of lung cancer, metastasized to the brain. He smoked lung-ripping Gauloises; and when I see someone remove one of those elegant periwinkle-blue packets of Gauloises from his pocket, I think of my friend Martin.

I often think of my friend Erich when the name of the brutish football coach Mike Ditka is mentioned. Erich, a Czech émigré and a scholar of Continental literature, whom illness forced to retreat into a retirement home, once asked me, in his Mitteleuropean-accented English, "Joe, who is dis man Ditka?" Erich, who used to sit in his small apartment reading Goethe and Rilke, and now living among old American men who talked lots of sports at meals, felt he had also to acquire knowledge of Ditka. "Erich," I told him, "he was a football player and once coach of the Chicago Bears, and there is no more you need ever know about him."

Whenever I hear an upper-class New York accent, I think of Fred, who began as one of my editors and ended as my friend. He was born wealthy, and lived well, though never piggishly, and had a splendid appetite for life. He had buried three children and known much deep sadness, which he never allowed to show through his regular spiritual uniform of bonhomie. He was also a good foxhole friend, Fred; once, when I was publicly attacked, he rushed to my defense with a strong letter to the *New York Times,* a letter of the kind that could have cost him favor with the forces of false virtue. He was a courageous and gracious man, and knowing he liked you gave you a higher opinion of yourself.

My friend Sam, who died just before he was sixty, of leukemia, used to call me at odd hours, which means he did so whenever the mood struck him, or when he had used up other friends, or when he couldn't, at the moment, find anyone more interesting to talk to. I assume there must have been days when he called one friend after another, pumping them for information, jokes, gossip, anything to keep his churning brain occupied. I didn't mind being used as a momentary stay against his boredom, which could be powerful and needed to be relieved. He had enormous energy, a perfervid imagination, and an overheated interest in the low side of politics. (How Sam would have loved the Bill Clinton and Monica Lewinsky scandal, I often thought during the year it clogged everyone's mind, but alas, he did not live to see it.)

During these phone conversations, which could last forty-five minutes or more, you could also feel Sam's interest in you begin to fade. When he had used you up, there would be a brief pause, and "OK" (pronounced *hoke-ay*), he would say, "talk to ya," and hang up. My wife and I have now adopted Sam's *hoke-ay,* which we use with each other whenever we feel we've exhausted a topic or one of us must depart. "*Hoke-ay,*" I say, and think: It is now more than ten years since I last heard Sam say it.

Some dead friends continue to exert an influence on the living. Edward Shils continues to have this beyond-the-grave influence on me. One of his self-appointed functions as a friend was that of unofficial conscience. He didn't exert it regularly on me, but he would call it into play from time to time. I remember once telling him that I was writing an essay on the poet Elizabeth Bishop, and his remarking that I really oughtn't to be wasting my time on such a slight subject. (Edward was, in cultural and intellectual matters, inimitably highbrow.) Occasionally I find myself doing things — watching two pro football games back to back or wasting an evening on a stupid movie — and I feel relieved that Edward is not around to ask me what I did yesterday or last night. Occasionally, too, I find myself saying things that seem to come from him, as if I were no more than a ventriloquist's dummy through whom he speaks from beyond the grave: "Harry Lester is the kind of nouveau riche who buys an extra box seat for his wife's hat" is something I said not long ago that could as easily — and probably a touch better — have been said by Edward. It's rather as if he is haunting me, but in a most entertaining way.

When I read the following "Greek Epigram," here rendered into English by William Johnson Cory, I thought immediately of my dear friend Edward:

> *They told me, Heraclitus, they told me you were dead,*
> *They brought me bitter news to hear, and bitter tears to shed.*
> *I wept as I remembered how often you and I*
> *Had tired the sun with talking and sent him down the sky.*
> *And now that thou art lying, my dear old Carian guest,*
> *A handful of grey ashes, long, long ago at rest,*
> *Still are thy pleasant voices, thy nightingales, awake;*
> *For Death, he taketh all away, but them he cannot take.*

The dead, if they made a strong impress upon us when they were alive, never leave us, not really, not finally.

The older one gets, obviously, the smaller the number of one's friends, unless one has invested in what the sociologists call "social capital," or the steady building up of friendships with people younger than oneself, people who, if one lives longer than one's contemporaries, will be around as friends. Samuel Johnson remarked that, upon the completion of his long-awaited edition of Shakespeare, he regretted that most of the people he "wished to please [with it] have sunk into the grave." Johnson was only forty-six when he expressed this sentiment. Despite the display of gloom, Johnson was, it must be said, adept at acquiring social capital, and did so consciously, writing to Sir Joshua Reynolds that "if a man does not make new acquaintance as he advances through life, he will soon find himself left alone."

The condition of friendlessness is one of life's sadnesses. So much of modern literature seems to be played out against such a condition: no friends in the works of Kafka, for example, and certainly none in that of Samuel Beckett. Most of Joseph Conrad's protagonists are friendless—it is what makes them so poignant, but also majestic. Conrad himself, though friendly in his manner, seemed to long for friendship in his own often difficult life. He is the author, after all, of "Amy Foster," perhaps the most powerful short story ever written on the theme of friendlessness.

The great novel of friendlessness is of course *Robinson Crusoe,* which I've recently read for the first time. (It is one of those novels that one thinks one has read, even if one hasn't; *1984* is another.) Many things make Daniel Defoe's a great book, and nothing at all of the children's book it is usually taken to be. But the most memorable thing about it is not so much how Crusoe masters his primitive environment by becoming a tolerably good farmer, herder, potter, butcher, carpenter, tailor, and much more, but how his survives his ordeal of utter loneliness.

In the book, Crusoe spends fully twenty-five years alone on the island before he saves his man Friday from cannibalism and has a companion at last. Perhaps no greater plea for the need for friendship has ever been written, for not even God, to whom Crusoe frequently talks—offering his thanks for the providential good luck of his life following the wretched luck of his originally having been a castaway—is a replacement for companionship. Through the first two-thirds of the book, Crusoe hints of his longings for a friend, and at one point he risks his own life, rowing out to another shipwreck in dangerous waters, in the hope of finding relief in the form of "somebody to speak to" on "this island of solitariness." His talking parrot, his dog, his domesticated cats, none can slacken his longing for "the comfort which the conversation that one of my fellow-Christians would have been to me."

The amiable Friday is not, of course, a Christian. He is, in fact, a cannibal, but he is human, and that is sufficient. The relation between the two men is one of master and servant, but the feeling between them is real; Friday is a man of good heart and honorable sentiment, and his example is such as to allow Crusoe to remark:

> This frequently gave me occasion to observe, and that with wonder, that however it had pleased God, in his providence and in the government of the works of his hands, to take from so great a part of the world of his creatures the best uses to which their faculties and the powers of their souls are adapted; yet that he has bestowed upon them the same powers, the same reason, the same affections, the same sentiments of kindness and obligation, the same passions and resentments of wrongs, the same sense of gratitude, sincerity, fidelity, and all the capacities of doing good and receiving good, that he has given to us, and that when he pleases to offer to them occasions of exerting these, they are as ready, nay, more ready, to apply them to the right uses for which they were bestowed than we are.

Once Crusoe teaches Friday to speak English — "he was the aptest scholar there ever was" — he has a friend, and his life now alters radically for the better. Above all, he is no longer alone. He calls the first year in the company of Friday "the pleasantest year of all the life I led in this place," and later adds that "the three years we lived there together [were] perfectly and completely happy, if any such thing as complete happiness can be formed in a sublunary state." Friendship, in other words, changes everything.

I have myself been notably friendless only for two short periods in my life. As a small boy, I was part of a crowd of kids but without any real friends of my own, this chiefly because I lived on a big-city block where almost all the other kids were older than I. My only brother was five and a half years younger than I, and thus, at that age, unqualified for friendship. I met kids at school I thought attractive, but I drew close to none of them. My life was lived on the block, and though I was at best a minor player there, I don't remember minding long stretches of solitude, a good deal of it spent listening to after-school and Saturday morning radio adventure shows.

Our family moved the summer I was ten, and the only kid on our block was a boy my age who turned out to be from an anti-Semitic family and was himself a pretty good Jew hater. I remember spending most of that summer on roller skates, the kind that one fit and tightened with a key, striding up and down the quiet street on which we now lived. Again, I cannot recall feeling any deep loneliness or social pain of any kind.

At what was to be my second grammar school, playing among kids my own age, I was considered a good athlete, which means my friendless days were over. Mine was a playground life, and I was among those early chosen for pickup games of various kinds. Being at or near the center of things carried over through high school, where I was a less notable athlete but, as I earlier recounted, a master of the delicate arts of conformity, the socially subtle operator pretty near par excellence.

The next time I can recall loneliness was when I was twenty-two and in the army, stationed in Little Rock, working at a recruiting station where my job was typing up physical examinations. Because there was no army base nearby, I was allowed to live in civilian conditions in an apartment of my own. Good duty, this was called in the army of those days, but it was also lonely duty. I would occasionally go for drinks with my fellow soldiers after a day at the recruiting station, but my nights and weekends were spent alone. Because we were overstaffed and the flow of recruits coming through the station varied greatly, I was often told to knock off at 11 A.M. for the day.

I had by then acquired a taste for books, and so I spent a fair amount of time alone in my furnished apartment reading books that I had borrowed from the main branch of the Little Rock library. Three hours was about the limit of my stamina for a session with a book. I would go out for long walks. At one point, I went to Sears and bought a basketball, and dribbled it for a few blocks to shoot a hundred free throws on a netless basket in a nearby schoolyard. I had no television, no radio. I would go to the movies occasionally, read the then quite good local paper (the *Arkansas Gazette*). Sometimes on a Saturday afternoon I would take myself to a nearby restaurant, order a beer at the bar, and watch a college football game.

"All the misfortunes of men derive from one single thing," wrote Pascal, "which is their inability to be at ease alone in a room." Pascal was correct about this, but did he also know that sitting in a room alone for a long stretch is much easier said than done? Rather than endure my sweet solitude, I began a quiet but sedulous pursuit of women, and then married one of those women I thought I had ensnared. As our living together for slightly less than a decade was to determine, she was the wrong woman, or perhaps I was the wrong man. Would this have happened in Chicago, where I would have been surrounded by lots of friends? Even though I thought myself a young man with what used to be called "inner resources," did I make this mistake owing to an inability to deal with solitude? Oh, Père Blaise, where were you with your good advice when I needed it?

Some rare people choose friendlessness, especially later in life. In a story called "Sail Shining in White," Mark Helprin has a character, an extremely self-reliant man, who sailed around the world alone more than once, and who, now in his early eighties, decides that he doesn't require friends.

He was without question an old man, but he did not carry his money in a clip, he had never had to give up golf (never having played it), and he neither watched nor owned a television. This, in conjunction with other things, meant that he had no friends. But he didn't want friends, because it was over, or just about to be over, and in preparing for the greatest moment alone he did not want shuffleboard, crafts, dinner theater, book discussions or college courses. He wanted, rather, to probe with a piecing eye to see in nature some clue to the mystery to come and the mysteries he would be leaving behind. He wanted a long and strenuous exercise of memory to summon in burning detail what he had loved. He wanted to bless, purify, and honor it, for if in the end he did not, he would by default have dishonored it.

In a Paul Simon song, old friends spend their days sitting on a park bench like bookends. Stray newspaper falls on the round toes of these old friends' high shoes, but more important for you to know is that these duffers are all of seventy, which now seems pretty damn young. (Paul Simon is himself today eligible for Social Security.)

But what makes this simple song poignant is the notion propelling it of dwindling friendship in old age. The choices aren't as stark, of course, as those offered between Mark Helprin's impressive fictional character and Paul Simon's befuddled old-timers. Old friends, like clear vision and quick reflexes, are among the losses of those who live into their eighties and nineties.

The poet John Frederick Nims was not a close, but I always felt a good, friend of mine — good in the sense that I was always pleased to see him, and I like to think he felt the same about me — of whose age I was never certain. He had kept his hair, and not much of it had turned gray. His personal style was whimsical; though his gravity was never in doubt, in conversation he kept things light. I assumed that John was in his seventies. When he died, his obituary in the *New York Times* gave his age as eighty-five.

When I asked John's wife how he had managed to seem not so much young as ageless, she revealed that his secret was never to talk about the past. Once one does talk about the past — that is, about one's own past — it almost invariably proves to be much better than the present. Castigate the present, and — ho, presto! — one is instantly an old-timer, crank division. Taking my lead from John Nims, I now try to evade talking about the past, except when in company made up exclusively of my contemporaries. Talking about this common past happens to give much pleasure, and what makes the elderly always a little sad is that, even on the Nimsian plan, they have fewer and fewer friends left to talk with about it.

Aristotle, in the *Nichomachean Ethics,* notes that "neither old nor sour people make friends easily." And yet new friendships acquired latish in life are always possible. I have made a few important friendships in my sixties, and am still hopeful about discovering others. To assume that no new friendships are possible would be to close down a significant part of one's life, and this must not be permitted.

If inspiration for beginning late-life friendships is needed, it is provided by a slender book called *A Late Friendship: The Letters of Karl Barth and Carl Zuckmayer.* Barth was the famous Swiss theologian, Zuckmayer the Austrian playwright and author of *Part of Myself,* a beautiful autobiographical volume. Both men of high Teutonic culture, each was already established in his fame when they met; Barth was eighty-one, Zuckmayer seventy. They met only three times, and mainly exercised their friendship through correspondence. Their full friendship extended just beyond a year, when Barth died at eighty-two.

The friendship began with a letter in June 1967 from Barth to Zuckmayer, congratulating him on a recent book of stories. The letter much pleased Zuckmayer by its warmth, lucidity, and understanding of his work. The two men met not long afterward; candor was immediate, confidences were exchanged. They found they could amiably disagree on subjects, though always with an overlay of what Zuckmayer called "a deep, basic agreement" on important things.

Such criticism as is exchanged between the two men mainly comes from Barth to Zuckmayer. Barth felt that Mozart was sublime among all composers, that Schubert, whom Zuckmayer loved, was limited by his Romanticism, and that Beethoven's grandest music proceeded not "from a liberated heart but a tortured mind." Barth lightly disputes Zuckmayer's saying that Frederick the Great was the most intelligent of monarchs, to which Zuckmayer rejoins that he should have said not the most intelligent but "the most cultured." Barth tells Zuckmayer that, though he realizes it is scarcely for him to say, perhaps it is a mistake for Zuckmayer to work on a play about the plot of the German generals to assassinate Hitler, for such material does not lend itself well to his talent, nor is the German-speaking public just now interested in such things. Zuckmayer accepts this in good part, and later concedes Barth was correct.

Barth and Zuckmayer were both earnest in their Christianity. Neither thought that the physical sciences came near explaining the mysteries of the world. They discussed changes in the Catholic Mass. Each had a strong taste for serenity, and a perspective that allowed them to consider all matters *sub specie aeternitatis,* or in the light of eternity.

Both knew the worth of public acclaim, which was pleasant but not to be taken all that seriously. When Barth congratulates Zuckmayer for winning an award, he also mentions an award recently given to him, then adds: "We are both people, are we not, who can have a good laugh at such things." Despite his age and his various illnesses, Barth continues to work. He cites Pablo Casals, then in his nineties, who, when asked why he continues to practice four or five hours a day, replies: "Because I believe I am making progress." Zuckmayer responds that he cannot imagine Barth not working.

Like any two older men, they have in common the grotesque comedy of their bodies shutting down on them. Barth refers to his ailments as events "unavoidably controlled by the less honorable members of my body." Zuckmayer has bladder and kidney problems, but they do not prevent him from working, as he puts it, "cheerfully." He allows that he has no plans to follow a nurse's advice to cut down on drinking and smoking, which might improve his blood pressure and circulation, because he feels that he then might "be too healthy, and that seems dangerous in old age." Barth, who was never without his lit pipe and had a passion for white wines, concurs, saying that the body mustn't be denied all it fancies.

Had Barth lived longer, he and Carl Zuckmayer might have formed one of those ideal friendships that Aristotle described millennia before: a friendship between two men of virtue, each of whom leads the other onto still higher paths of virtue. Might it be that, in our time, one has to arrive at an advanced age before one can hope to acquire the wisdom needed for such a friendship? It might well, though one would prefer serene friendships to begin much earlier in life, if only so that the deep pleasure they yield may be enjoyed longer.

# 19

❖

# *Is There an Art of Friendship?*

WHEN I FIRST SET OUT to write a book on friendship, I began with a vague sense that the standard idealization of friends was somehow false to the truth of friendship, at least as, day by day, we all live it. I also sensed my own slight discomfort at sometimes being put off by the mild but often insistent demands of friends, though I enjoyed being with my friends and think myself a friendly person. I recognized that I was promiscuous in my friendships, and would sometimes feel trapped in a friendship I hadn't really wanted. For reasons that were less than clear to me, what was supposed to have been one of life's pure pleasures had become complicated and sometimes confused.

Friendship, I came to realize, ought not to be considered so free and easy a thing as it generally is, but needs to be treated as an art. Like any other art, it requires perspective, craft, a careful and experienced touch. It calls for regular maintenance through thoughtful cultivation. To know oneself is the first and best step in the training for friendship, and from there one hopes to go on to know one's friends. In friendship the golden rule — treat others as you would yourself be treated — doesn't always apply. Some friends, after all, wish to be treated quite differently than one wishes to be treated oneself. But treating friendship as an art, and not as a series of social accidents or spontaneous happenings, is essential.

The very word friendship, like stewardship, editorship, governorship, and several other words with a *-ship* suffix, implies not passivity but an active hand; it suggests taking control, charting a course, planning a future. Most of us, I suspect, do not look upon friendship in this way. Until writing this book, I certainly didn't. Instead I took my friends as they came. Some have been a continuing delight to me, some have seemed burdensome, some I regret ever having started up with and, given the opportunity, would prefer to trade away for players to be named later.

"The name of friend seems to me even holier [than that of relative]," wrote Quintilian, the first-century Roman advocate. "For the one comes from the intellect, comes from a decision; the other chance bestows, circumstance of birth and things that are not elected by our will." Quintilian is correct when he says that one's friends are a matter of conscious decision. True, sometimes one's choices are limited by circumstances. But if many of one's friends seem given, like cards dealt out, perhaps one does best to think of the game of friendship as five-card draw, in which one can toss away some cards and ask for others. One doesn't have to stick with the hand one was dealt.

Only of late have I begun to become more selective, in effect to attempt to edit my friendships. I not long ago learned that the mother of my physician died. He is a man I like; we have long called each other by first names. It occurred to me to send him a note of condolence, but then I thought better of it. Such a note might draw us closer together. But is more closeness needed? Our middle-distance friendship seems fine as it is. I'm certain he doesn't want more closeness from me. I decided not to send the note.

The columnist George Will occasionally calls me when he is in Chicago, where he has a son and grandchildren living. Sometimes we go to lunch or dinner together; he recently took me to a Cubs game, treating me to a front-row seat. Soon after, I happened to read an interesting article on the relief pitcher Dennis Eckersley in *GQ*, which I'm fairly certain he doesn't read. I cut it out of the magazine intending to send it to him, then decided not to do so. Why put him under the obligation of having to read it, write to me about it, perhaps call to tell me an odd fact or two (he has a vast quantity of such facts) about Eckersley. I like the occasional nature of my friendship with George, who is a man much on the go, and see no reason to take it any further or deepen it in any way. It's quite all right as it is.

I have developed a taste for highly qualified, nicely defined friendships — the equivalent, I suppose, of prenuptial agreements but applied to friends. I have a friend who lives in Arizona and who, on his annual visit to Chicago, meets me for a single lunch. I see another friend perhaps four or five times a year, always for coffee. I once suggested that we get together with our wives, but there were complications on his side in doing so. I have not suggested it again. Things are OK as they are, I have decided, and I shall not again suggest meeting with wives.

A man who lived in the same apartment building I do went to my high school four years before I did. We had had many acquaintances in common. A year or so ago, he died, of a heart attack, while out exercising on his bicycle. Ours was largely an elevator and lobby friendship. I was always pleased to see him, and I like to think he felt the same about me. We were never without things to tell each other: news of old schoolmates, fresh jokes, chitchat about sports. I don't believe that we ever had a conversation lasting beyond twenty minutes. I could have invited him to lunch, where with more time our friendship might have become richer, but I never did. Nor did he ever invite me to lunch; a wise man, perhaps he instinctively understood the art of friendship without first having to write an entire book on the subject. The first rule of the art of friendship, I have come to believe, is that not all friendships need to be deepened.

Another rule I have devised is never to allow friendship to be reduced to a sharing of afflictions; friendship oughtn't to consist mainly, or even secondarily, of sharing weaknesses or troubles. One mustn't unload, as we say nowadays, on one's friends one's terrors, disappointments, and (until now hidden) resentments at the world's putative injustices. The art of friendship entails deliberate repression. A friend, a cliché definition has it, is someone who, when you are in crisis, you can call at 4 A.M. I'd say that's true, but with the qualification that one is permitted only one such call.

Yet another rule of the art of friendship is to look beyond the mere opinions of potential friends in the attempt to discover that deeper thing, their point of view. Everyone has opinions, lots of them, but not everyone has a point of view, which is much more than the collectivity of a person's opinions. A point of view is one's particular angle on the world, one's ways of viewing life that imply a well-considered position on a range of much larger questions than that of the reform of Social Security or the future of NATO. Not everyone has a point of view; one perhaps has to reach a certain maturity to develop one. But those who have reached chronological maturity and still haven't done so are unlikely to make good friends, at least not for people who consider themselves thoughtful.

I am myself guilty of breaking a serious rule of the art of friendship, the Aristotelian stricture against *polyphilia*, or having too many friends: "for it would seem," Aristotle wrote, "actually impossible to be a great friend to many people." In a talk I once gave on friendship, I mentioned that I have seventy-five or so friends. A sensible woman in the audience said that that seemed an unusually, almost unbelievably, high number. (I'm reminded here of reading somewhere that William F. Buckley, Jr., once gave a party to which he invited his fifteen hundred closest friends.) I now think that the number seventy-five was probably on the modest side, at least if one thinks of friends as people with whom one has had past and expects to have continuing relations, with all the conviviality and obligations entailed in a friendship. Doubtless it is now too late, but if I could, I shouldn't mind cutting down my roster of friends. On the other hand, if I had had a severely limited number of friends, I might not have been able to write this book.

Part of the art of friendship, I have also decided, includes reassessing the pleasures of acquaintanceship, which may be underrated. I once thought I would have a chapter in this book called "Let Old Acquaintance Be Forgot," but I've come to think there is much to be said on behalf of acquaintances, not least the absence of obligation that they bring. In *Snobs,* Julian Fellowes, through his narrator, who is an actor, offers several kind words for acquaintanceship, which he claims to prefer over close friendship: "I am an observer. It troubles me to be forced into the role of participant."

Friendship requires participation. Not all fields of endeavor permit the time that full participation in friendship requires. The choice of being an artist, which is to say an observer, greatly reduces the appetite for frequent engagements with friends. From Thoreau to James Joyce, from Tolstoy to Samuel Beckett, from Melville to Saul Bellow, literary artists, while not without friends, have never been notable for devoting much energy to the enterprise of friendship. (Nor, from Napoleon to Bismarck to Franklin Delano Roosevelt to Winston Churchill, have great political figures done much better.) "Friends are a costly luxury," wrote Ibsen. "When a man invests his capital of energy in a profession or mission, he will lack the means to have friends."

Her biographer Richard Sewall wrote of Emily Dickinson that "she never achieved a single, wholly satisfying relationship with anybody she had to be near, or with, for any length of time." Henry James was kind and generous to many people, but his first obligation was to his art. One of his biographers writes about Isaac Bashevis Singer that he "was a consummate master of casual acquaintance," which is another way of saying that he knew how to keep people at a proper distance. Celeste Alberet, Marcel Proust's housekeeper, in her memoir of her employer, writes "that he must have let, or even made, a lot of people think he felt affection and friendship for them, whereas in fact — it was the thing that always struck me — he could do without all of them with the greatest ease."

One finds such coolness over and over in artists. In a song called "Being Alive," the finale to his show *Company,* Stephen Sondheim writes of a close friend that he may be someone you need too much and you know too well, someone who'll put you through hell. For all their astonishing gifts, Michelangelo, Mozart, Beethoven, Dostoyevsky, and Picasso seem not to have had much of a gift for friendship. The last great modernist artist, the choreographer George Balanchine, who had five wives, seems to have had fewer friends. Loyal and generous though he was to the people in his great dance company, "he was a person you could not get close to," as one of his male dancers remarked. "We never got to feel 'this is my friend.'" Balanchine himself said, "I can't cope with human relationships, difficult relationships." His art, the reason surely is, came first.

Dorothy Rowe, an Australian writer and psychotherapist, in a book titled *Friends and Enemies,* asked a number of people who participated in various workshops she ran to end a sentence that began, "After it's all said and done, what matters most in life is . . ." The four things that were most often listed were "a sense of having achieved something"; "a sense of having made a contribution to the world"; "being able to accept yourself and so be at peace with yourself"; and "loving relationships." She notes: "What was listed most often was loving relationships. What most people feared was dying unloved and alone."

My guess is that most artists would have written one of the first two responses, and the more passionate they were about their art, the less that the last one was likely to have entered into their thinking. In the division of people between those who live for their work and those who work chiefly in order to live, artists fall preponderantly on the live-to-work side. Alexis de Tocqueville, despondent at the end of his active political career, writes: "For without the resource of a great book to write, I truly do not know what would become of me." People who are more devoted to the pleasures of daily life are likely to be more intensely interested in the cultivation of friendship.

One of the toughest rules of the art of friendship is to take friends as they are. It hasn't always been easy for me to do so. I have a strong critical sense, with a passion for analysis, and an abiding interest in the motives, known and secret, of others, not least those of my friends. I feel a need to understand—not do anything about, but merely understand—the vanities and weaknesses of friends along with their virtues and strengths. I want to know what movie is playing in their minds in which they think they have a starring role. Such a need is not, to reverse the cant phrase, user-friendly. I earlier quoted Samuel Johnson advising that we "take friends such as we find them, not as we would make them." I believe I am willing to take friends as I find them, but only after taking the most precise measure of them possible, so I have a strong sense of who, exactly, they are.

The art of friendship involves knowing what you want, need, expect, and are willing to give to other people in a friendship. In late middle age, what I most want from friends is amusingly engaging talk. From some people, I have come to expect talk that cuts deeper than it does from others. Although such talk can be quite enough, I also hope that sometimes my friends will cause me to discover things about myself and the world that, without their intervention, I would never have discovered on my own. In recompense, I hope I can sometimes do something similar for them through such insights and observations and amusements as I might have to bestow.

Friends have conferred favors on me. One friend regularly bails me out of small computer problems, sometimes at the cost of nearly a full day of work; another often calls bits of journalism and scholarship to my attention that I might not otherwise have known about; yet another, a woman who goes to house sales, keeps an eye out for things that she thinks might charm me: a pair of unused dove-gray spats is one recent delightful gift of hers in this line.

I also obtain from friends an unacknowledged reinforcement of my belief in my own worth. I am more than a little pleased, for example, to think that I have become friendly with most of the men and women I admire who work in the realms of art and intellect. This suggests that they may also have some tincture of admiration for me and what I do, which of course delights me.

Mine has been a lucky enough life for me not to need to call upon friends for loans of money, or the gift of bone marrow or a kidney, or much in the way of emotional support. I have a friend who recently wrote to me in the most heartfelt way about the death of a friend of his who was immensely helpful to him when his, my friend's, wife was undergoing something close to a nervous breakdown and he had no one in his own family to talk with about his troubles; and he did something similar when this man's own wife died. "No matter how stupid or crass or idiotic they may occasionally be, friends are friends," he wrote to me shortly after this man had died. They are, he said, "the people you connect with."

As for what I expect from friends, I mainly expect consideration, which includes a set of reasonably correct assumptions about the sort of man I am. A friend ought to know something about how another friend's mind works, how his tastes run, what he finds amusing, and what intolerable.

In the line of expectations, friends ought to be able to ask friends favors. The extent of the favors, however, is what is in question. I am up for doing any favors I can for friends. I am ready to use such connections as I have to help friends, or the children or cousins of friends, find editorial jobs and literary agents, or offer advice on their careers. I stand prepared to drive friends wherever they need to go. I have loaned some friends small sums, never more than a thousand dollars.

Favors in friendship need to be carefully calibrated. Aristotle said that no friend should ever ask one to do anything that is (morally) wrong. But at a level below the moral, things get more complicated. In a *Seinfeld* episode, Jerry meets the Mets' first baseman Keith Hernandez, who soon thereafter asks Jerry if he would help him move his furniture into a new apartment. A subtle, convoluted, and amusing discussion follows among Jerry's friends about the appropriateness of the request, given that the two men have known each other so brief a time; the point is that the favor, given the short acquaintanceship between the two men, seems out of line.

Sometimes a favor will be offered that one hadn't expected and is so delighted by that one looks upon the person bestowing it in an entirely different way. One evening, setting out for a concert, our car didn't start. A neighbor, with whom I had previously done nothing more than exchange polite greetings, noting my problem, without hesitation offered me the use of his car for the evening. I was much impressed by the offer, which I gratefully took him up on. The generosity of the gesture moved him for me out of the mere neighbor category. We were talking the other day about the agreeable way that the people in our building keep a proper distance from one another. I agreed that this was so, adding only that he and I were in serious danger of becoming friends. He smiled.

A generous impulse ought never to be stifled, or so I have always felt. But if friendship is to be practiced artfully, even generosity may sometimes have to be measured. (Benjamin Franklin, that genius of the practical, once said that the way to win a person over is not to do favors for him but to arrange to have him do a favor for you. After he has done so, he will always look upon you benignly, as a person he has helped through life, a living symbol of his own magnanimity.) Overkill may occur; how, one wonders, will one ever be able to square things, put them back on a fair basis, so that a favor doesn't come to take the form of an obligation? Sometimes you can do a friend a real favor by not doing him too great a favor.

Perhaps the first rule in the art of friendship is never to idealize a friend. A friend is not a dog, a Lassie, a Benjy, a Rin Tin Tin, a permanently affectionate, unconditionally loving creature offering uncritical adoration and someone who is always going to come through for you. Owing to such general idealization, altogether too much pressure is placed on friendship, with the result that one comes to expect perfection, which isn't likely to be available even in the best of friends. Friends, in fact, figure to be unsteady, contradictory, not perpetually obliging — rather, if I may say so, like you and, it pains me much more to say, like me.

If one had to draw a brief character of the author of this book, it might well be that he is a gregarious melancholic, a highly sociable misanthrope, a laughing skeptic. On different days, or on the same day, he is distinctly more or less hospitable to the delights and obligations of friendship, welcoming it warmly one day, doing very nicely without it, thank you very much, the next. Life without friends is unimaginable, but life with them perpetually around is no picnic on the grass, either.

The idealization of friendship may be owing to the fact that the most intense time for friendship, for men and women, is during adolescence. This is also a period when time itself seems inexhaustible, and life's pressures are well off in the distance. Friendship can be explored, friends cultivated, unambiguously enjoyed, luxuriated in.

My own adolescence, I see now, was devoted wholly to friendship. Each morning I thought of myself as going off not to school, in which my interest wasn't even minimal, but to the prospect of exchanges with a wide circle of friends, close, middle-distance, and happily negligible friends. Every day was spent at play in the fields of friends, bopping from circle to circle of pals in gym, at the school store where we all gathered at lunch and after school, and usually continuing through the evening, with time out only for dinner at home, laughing and splashing my way through the day in the warm waters of friendship. I am supposed, I believe, to regret this extended frivolousness. It was a thorough waste of time, during which I could have learned ancient Greek or taken up the oboe; it was completely irresponsible; it was paradise.

Not that friendship is one of those childish things that must be put away once one attains adulthood, or that one must henceforth view it, as the First Epistle to the Corinthians says, through a glass, darkly. But life contrives many ways of pushing friendship off center stage the older one grows. From its high point in adolescence, it tends to descend in centrality next to marriage, family, passion for work, and sometimes, too, with a heightened consciousness of the rush of time passing.

Enough has changed over the past fifty or so years to alter the nature of friendship substantially. Begin with the changed status of women. As we have seen in the classical writers, wives in the good/bad old days were generally not considered candidates for friendship with their husbands. Until the advent of labor-saving devices such as washers and dryers, only aristocratic or wealthy women had much time for friendships of their own, even with other women. The emergence of women in the workplace, with the greater affluence and freedom it has sometimes brought them, has changed much about friendship, not least the old strict division into exclusively male and female friends.

The phenomenon of women out working in the world has obviously changed the way the family works, and with it the older formation of friendships. The family is now a less tightly controlled ship than it was when one person (the wife and mother) was at the wheel. Men are now called upon to help out, and are fools if they don't agree to do so. With both parents often working, the feeling of frenzy, even when there is increased income to buffer it, is fairly standard. Add to all this the frequency of divorce, which can lend the leaden note of guilt to that of frenzy.

This feeling of frenzy has a good deal to do with the heavily increased amount of attention that children now receive. Most homes with young kids today are child-centered to an extent that would astonish parents of my mother and father's generation, who brought up their children in the 1940s and '50s. Neither of my parents felt that their first duty was to their children. They went off on vacations to Montreal or New York and left my younger brother and me in the care of professional babysitters or a childless aunt and uncle. My mother didn't begin driving until her late forties, and my father was always off at work during the day, including Saturday, so I was never picked up or taken anywhere by my parents; I bicycled or took public transportation wherever I went. True, the world seemed a safer place then — less crime, no drugs — and kids could be left on their own more readily. But I never felt in the least neglected or maltreated by being so much on my own; on the contrary, I relished the freedom. Few parents today would themselves feel free enough to extend such freedom to their own children. Such is their worry about bringing up their children properly that they are willing (feel compelled is more like it) to expend a vast outlay of time on a full-court press of attention for their kids — time taken from, among other things, the cultivating of friendships.

Given the changed status of women, the demands of career and especially those of family in the contemporary scheme of living, friendship has been demoted to a leisure time activity and consequently has come to seem an altered, even a radically changed, institution.

At moments in the course of writing this book I had the staggering thought that I seemed to be coming out against friendship — turning out one of those drab volumes carrying a title like *The Death of Friendship*. That is not at all what I had in mind when I began, and it is not what I have ended up with. What I wanted was to take some of the air out of the idealization of friendship, so that a friend, like a teacher or a clergyman, need not always feel that he or she is falling short of an impossible ideal.

Friendship is often an amusement, sometimes an education, at least a reprieve from loneliness, at best a human connection of the highest and grandest kind. Contradiction is implicit in the very nature of modern friendship. F. Scott Fitzgerald said that the sign of an intelligent person is the ability to keep two contradictory ideas in his head at the same time and still function. With friendship, the two contradictory ideas are these: first, friends can be an immense complication, a huge burden, and a royal pain in the arse; and, second, without friendship, make no mistake about it, we are all lost.

*A Bibliographical Note*

*Acknowledgments*

*Index*

# A Bibliographical Note

This is not a book built on other books. Not that there haven't been fine books built on other books, but on the subject of friendship the books aren't there, at least not yet, or at any rate not enough of them of sufficient quality on which to build.

Certainly there isn't that one usually large, splendidly comprehensive book that one sometimes encounters on other subjects. I not long ago wrote a little book on the subject of envy and discovered a book of the kind I have in mind called *Envy: A Theory of Social Behavior* by Helmut Schoeck. More recently I was asked to give a lecture on the celebrity culture and discovered a splendid history of fame called *The Frenzy of Renown: Fame and Its History* by Leo Braudy. These are books whose authors, having thoroughly worked up their subjects, did all the heavy lifting of research and cleared away the debris for writers who come after them.

On the subject of friendship there is no such book. (Nor is the volume in your hands such a book, either. Writing such a book would require a far more diligent hand than my own.) After the twenty-odd pages of Aristotle in the *Nichomachean Ethics*, Cicero's fine essay *De Amicitia*, Montaigne's essay "On Friendship," one of the sections of C. S. Lewis's *Four Loves*, writings on friendship thin out fast. Some famous writers — Plato, Ralph Waldo Emerson, and a few others — are rather disappointing on the subject.

Sociology has come to study friendship only in recent decades. Ray Pahl, in *On Friendship*, has written a brief but excellent survey of the issues, questions, and problems friendship presents in its contemporary settings. Digby Anderson, in *Losing Friends,* examines the changing nature of friendships, which he does not think a good thing. Letty Cottin Pogrebin's *Among Friends* is a useful book written from a sensibly feminist perspective. The sociology of friendship tends to come at things at too high, too abstract, a level of generality. If the subject of friendship were a play, the sociology of it is still, one senses, at the point of moving furniture around the stage.

The best writers on friendship are novelists, though there are not, to my knowledge, all that many novels that take up the subject directly; a fine exception is William Maxwell's novel of adolescent friendship, *The Folded Leaf.* Friendship looms large in the work of E. M. Forster, and Charles Dickens is marvelous at conveying the warmth that honorable and selfless friendship can bring. *Robinson Crusoe* is the great work on friendlessness.

Good anthologies collecting poems, essays, and stories featuring friendship exist. *The Norton Book of Friendship* and *The Oxford Book of Friendship* are perhaps the best in this line. Collections of letters between friends nicely illustrate friendship in practice. More often than not, the best bits about friendship are to be found by the way, in aphorisms, in sentences plucked from novels, in the stray observations of such philosophers as Nietzsche and Santayana and Michael Oakeshott.

For all the reasons cited above, and for a few others, this book is built less on its author's reading and more on his personal experience. I hope that readers have not taken my writing so much about myself in its pages as pure, pushing egotism. My defense is similar to the one that Max Beerbohm, a writer I much admire, made to his wife for writing a good deal about himself:

> I am not thinking that "I am I" and must be interesting to everyone else. I am nothing more than I—a detached and puzzled spectator—detached, yet knowing more about myself than any other subject, and offering myself humbly for the inspection of others. I think there is a difference between this and egotism.

I do, too.

But here is a list of the books, some read through, some merely consulted, I found useful while working on *Friendship: An Exposé*.

Adams, Rebecca G., and Graham A. Allan, *Placing Friendship in Context*

Allan, Graham A., *A Sociology of Friendship and Kinship*

Anderson, Digby, *Losing Friends*

Aristotle, *Nichomachean Ethics*

Barth, Karl, and Carl Zuckmayer, *A Late Friendship: The Letters of Karl Barth and Carl Zuckmayer*, translated by Geoffrey W. Bromiley

Bate, W. Jackson, *Samuel Johnson*

Burke, Peter, *The Art of Conversation*

Colette, *Break of Day*

Defoe, Daniel, *Robinson Crusoe*

Duck, Steve, *Friends for Life*

Enright, D. J., and David Rawlinson, editors, *The Oxford Book of Friendship*

*The Epicurus Reader: Selected Writings and Testimonials*, translated and edited by Brad Inwood and L. P. Gerson

Everitt, Anthony, *Cicero: The Life and Times of Rome's Greatest Politician*

Fellowes, Julian, *Snobs*

Fischer, Claude S., *To Dwell Among Friends: Personal Networks in Town and City*

Forster, E. M., *Howards End*

Forster, E. M., *A Passage to India*

Freud, Sigmund, *The Complete Letters of Sigmund Freud to Wilhelm Fliess*, translated and edited by Jeffrey Moussaieff Masson

Gee, Lisa, *Friends: Why Men and Women Are from the Same Planet*

Haseldine, Julian, editor, *Friendship in Medieval Europe*

Hazlitt, William, *Collected Essays of William Hazlitt*

Herman, Gabriel, *Ritualised Friendship and the Greek City*

Konstan, David, *Friendship in the Classical World*

Lamb, Charles, *Essays of Elia*

Lewis, C. S., *The Four Loves*

Mann, Thomas, and Erich Kahler, *An Exceptional Friendship:
The Correspondence of Thomas Mann and Erich Kahler*

Martin, Robert Bernard, *With Friends Possessed: A Life of
Edward Fitzgerald*

Maxwell, William, *The Folded Leaf*

Miller, Stuart, *Men and Friendship*

Mitford, Nancy, and Evelyn Waugh, *The Letters of Nancy
Mitford and Evelyn Waugh,* edited by Charlotte Mosley

Monsour, Michael, *Women and Men as Friends: Relationships
Across the Life Span in the Twenty-first Century*

Nardi, Peter M., *Gay Men's Friendships*

Nietzsche, Friedrich, *The Gay Science*

Nietzsche, Friedrich, *Human, All Too Human*

O'Connor, Pat, *Friendships Between Women*

Oz, Amos, *A Tale of Love and Darkness*

Pahl, Ray, *On Friendship*

Pamuk, Orhan, *The White Castle*

Plato, *Dialogues of Plato*

Pogrebin, Letty Cottin, *Among Friends*

Porter, Roy, and Sylvana Tomaselli, *The Dialectics of
Friendship*

Rieff, Philip, *The Triumph of the Therapeutic*

Rowe, Dorothy, *Friends and Enemies*

Salamensky, S. I., editor, *Talk, Talk, Talk: The Cultural Life
of Everyday Conversation*

Simmel, Georg, *The Sociology of Georg Simmel,* translated,
edited, and with an introduction by Kurt H. Wolff

Taylor, A. E., *Epicurus*

Tiger, Lionel, *Men in Groups*

Welty, Eudora, and Ronald A. Sharp, editors, *The Norton Book
of Friendship*

Yager, Jan, *Friendshifts: The Power of Friendship and How It
Shapes Our Lives*

Yager, Jan, *When Friendship Hurts: How to Deal with Friends
Who Betray, Abandon, or Wound You*

# Acknowledgments

I owe a vast debt to Arnie Glass, to whom this book is dedicated. Not only did he suggest the idea for this book to me, but over the course of its composition he frequently talked with me about it and read various chapters with sympathy and penetration, always returning them to me with usefully provocative criticisms. I should also like to thank Webster Younce, the book's editor, for suggesting, with unfailingly witty and winning tact, many intelligent ways, small and large, to improve the original version of the book.

# Index